"Public Health Services for All": Revitalizing a Shattered Plan

Harold M. Erickson, Sr., M.D., M.P.H.

1993

ISBN 88-888-88888

Cover art by Andy Nelson
Book design and typesetting by Peregrine Publications

Acknowledgements and Thanks

To my dear wife who encouraged, supported, and assisted me during the many years of writing, revising, and editing this book.

To my sons, Harold M. Erickson, Jr., M.D., Donald K. Erickson, A.I.C.P., and Richard H. Erickson, for their suggestions and valuable assistance, and to Robert F. Erickson, M.D., and his wife, Sandra, who were very helpful in proof-reading and in arranging for publication.

I would like particularly to thank Donald A. Henderson, M.D., M.P.H. Dean emeritus, The Johns Hopkins University School of Hygiene and Public Health, for reading the manuscript, for his suggestions, and for his generous and heartening letters on the importance of the text.

To Wilson T. Sowder, M.D., M.P.H. who has been very supportive in his comments and in giving permission to share experiences as State Director of Health from his book "Florida's Health under Eleven Governors".

I appreciated the help that Malcolm H. Merrill, M.D., M.P.H., former State Director of Health of California, a great friend, gave me in reading an early version of the manuscript and in making suggestions for organizing and publishing. Likewise my thanks to Dr. Arthur Koski for his valuable suggestions, and to Paul Reid, D.D.S, M.P.H. and Edward B. Cowan, Jr., D.D.S. who reviewed the section on dental health.

Lee Cole, one of my outstanding secretaries did a superb job in typing the original manuscript and who has maintained her enthusiasm for publication of this book for many years. Jay Cole, her husband, was helpful in obtaining photographs and researching legislation on hospitals.

Thanks to my good friend, Ross Nichols, now over 100 years old, who shared experiences with me on early medical and hospital care; and to the Mary Hitchcock Memorial Center staff for photos of the original and of the new hospital.

A special thanks to my grandson, Colin Erickson, who edited the manuscript. He made valuable suggestions for revisions, deletions, illustrations, and for the cover.

Finally, I would express my appreciation to Margaret E. Mahoney, President, The Commonwealth Fund, Bert Kruger Smith, Hogg Foundation for Mental Health, Dr. Harold and Susan Osterud, and the many others who have helped with their suggestions.

Contents

Preface 1
1. Evolvement of Health Departments 6
   A. Early Leadership 10
   B. Plan for Local Health Units for the Nation 14
2. Crisis in Public Health 26
3. Record of Successes of Health Departments Combating Communicable Disease: 33
   A. Early Scourges 33
   B. Polio and Influenza 54
4. Health Department Contributions in Control of Sexually Transmitted Diseases 66
5. Role in Control of Tuberculosis 98
6. Attacking Other Threats to Public Health 109
7. Contributions in Control of Nutritional Deficiency Diseases 130
8. Better Health for Mothers, Infants, and Children 133
9. Mental Health Services 149
10. Transformation of Hospitals and Other Care Facilities 165
11. Preserving Our Teeth 182
12. Environmental Surveilance for Better Health 192
   A. Water Supplies 192
   B. Pollution Control 0
13. Bookkeeping of Humanity 212
14. Promoting Better Health 219
15. Public Health Nursing 226
16. Failure of Leaders 230
17. Excessive Involvement in Medical Care? 233
18. Inadequate Financing 236
19. Political Influence 242
20. Cost Effectiveness of Health Department Prevention Services 262
21. And What of the Future for "Local Health Units for the Nation" 264
References 273
About the Author 274

"A country with no regard for its past will do little worth remembering in the future."

Attributed to Abraham Lincoln

Preface

Preventive public health services are fragmented, inadequate, poorly distributed, and in many areas of the country in shambles, or non-existent. An excellent plan to develop a comprehensive service through "Local Health Units for the Nation" was developed in the thirties and early forties. Many successful Health departments, although short-staffed, were established as envisioned in the plan. Now the majority of these Health Departments are under-staffed, insufficiently financed, often over-whelmed with medical care responsibilities which have superceded vital health services of "prevention." Many departments are handicapped due to political interference, fragmentation of responsibility, and lack of competent leadership. The "Plan" was never fully implemented. Had it been, our preventive public health services, and our public health infrastructure, would not be in such chaos.

The intent of the plan was sound. Especially trained public health personnel including public health physicians, public health nurses, sanitarians, health educators, vital statisticians, laboratory staff, and clerical personnel, acting as a team and cooperating with private physicians, would assure that every person in this country would have the benefit of essential preventive health services. The beginnings of achieving the goal were encouraging. Thousands of public health physicians, public health nurses, and other vital public health personnel were trained and employed. Expectant mothers were being located early and brought under medical care. Infants, preschool, and school children were being immunized, given health exams, and disabilities corrected or cared for. Milk and water supplies were cleaned up. Water pollution, air pollution, and radiation control programs were initiated. Many communicable diseases were brought under control. The decline of community public health services began after major curtailment due to World War II. That deterioration, after an initial resurgence, has continued since due to any of a number of possible causes. Implementation of the "Plan" floundered and its objectives have never been achieved.

Why? Was the "Plan" unrealistic? What factors or influences brought about the present chaotic state of dwindling preventive public health services? Should it—and more realistically, can it—be revitalized and implemented?

As a participant in the early implementation of the plan and as a keenly interested observer, I saw many new Health Units being established, existing Health Departments expanded, and excellent public health services being provided with outstanding success, only to witness the gradual disintegration of these vital services in subsequent years. I firmly believe that recording many of my observations, analyzing developments, and the constructive influences as well as the destructive forces that impacted and prevented the realization of the "Plan", could be of significant value in re-vitalizing such a "Plan." In doing so, I would hope to acquaint the general public and to remind government officials of early threats to public health and of those successful public health programs established to attack and conquer them. I would like to explain how successful preventive public health services, in which Health Departments played a major role, were developed and how, excluding rhetoric, these services are now being neglected. I also would emphasize how these services have been fragmented, and in many cases destroyed due to wars, through various actions of the Congress, special interest influence, de-professionalization, loss of leadership, public unawareness of the facts and a general apathy.

My objective is to clarify the reasons for the failure to implement, not only the "Plan", but also other plans such as "Model Standards for Community Preventive Health Services." It is my hope that public recognition of the value of well-organized preventive health services and of how these services are being destroyed might lead to a public demand to reactivate the "Plan.'

As a young physician trained in pediatric surgery, I entered the field of public health indirectly as a product of the "Great Depression" years. Along with many other new, young physicians, I was given the opportunity to engage primarily in the practice of preventive medicine and public health. After seeing the great value of such services, I became enthusiastic about the potential for serving the public in this relatively new speciality. I gave up my career in pediatric surgery realizing that I could serve more people, save more lives, and prevent more illness in public health than I could as a surgeon.

I was fortunate in receiving an appointment as a local health officer to establish and direct an ideally staffed health department. This was in the Wasco and Sherman counties of Oregon in 1937. This department was unusual in that it provided primarily preventive health services. It did not engage in medical care except to treat patients with sexually transmitted disease (STD). The department cooperated fully with and had the support of the private physicians in the community. It could not have been successful otherwise. The Public Health Nurses (and Aides) served as an extended arm of the private physicians' offices. The Health Department located expectant mothers, infants, and children in need of care. Through personal conferences and health education they motivated them to see their own doctors. The latter provided the essential care.

Identifying needs without follow-up and medical care is fruitless. Clinics and individual physicians' services and health department staff services complement each other to assure good care. The health officer has as his patient the entire community. Just as the clinician examines, diagnoses, and treats the individual patient, the Health Officer and his staff, where adequate, diagnose the most serious community health problems and establish programs to resolve them.

After three years of service I was truly impressed with the dramatic reduction in maternal and infant deaths, in the reduction of cases of tuberculosis, smallpox, STD, and other communicable disease, and with improvements in general sanitation. In the Wasco and Sherman counties the department may have been new, but the improvement in the health of the community was readily apparent and was recognized nationally. Measures to clean up milk and water supplies, to bring restaurants up to Public Health Service standards (through grading), to control mosquitoes, rats, and ground squirrels, were very effective and were enthusiastically supported by the public. Similar progress was being made in many areas of the country.

Hopes were high. The plan for local health units for the nation was becoming a reality. Public health personnel across the nation received stipends made available by Congress for special training in public health and in public health administration. Universities established or expanded schools of Public Health with Federal aid. With this infusion of additional trained staff, the establishment of new health departments, as well as vitalizing and strengthening older ones, was made possible. The American Public

Health Association staff provided support to state health departments and local communities in organizing and establishing local health departments and services. The National Tuberculosis Association and state and local affiliates recognized the importance of local health departments in the control of tuberculosis. They gave immeasurable assistance in mobilizing community support for these services. Hundreds of local health departments were established bringing preventive health services never before experienced, to a significant portion of the nation's population with great success.

In 1937 the first of the National Institutes of Health, the National Cancer Institute, was created. This came about under the leadership of exceedingly well-qualified career United States Public Health Service (USPHS) physicians. On July 1, 1946, the Communicable Disease Center was officially established. These two facilities are now recognized throughout the world as unsurpassed health research centers. At this time there was a move to centralize National Health programs under the USPHS. Responsibility for Indian Health was transferred from the Bureau of Indian Affairs to the USPHS. Mental Health was established as one of its programs. Maternal and Child Health programs which had been administered by the Children's Bureau became a part of the USPHS, and many other programs including those for the prevention of heart disease, cancer, arthritis, diabetes, drug abuse, alcoholism, allergic and infectious disease and accidents were developed under the direction of the USPHS.

Concurrently state health department public health services expanded and extended under the guidance of able state boards of health. This occurred with the assistance of federal funds and with consultation from the USPHS and Children's Bureau.

With the outbreak of World War II it was necessary to divert staff from health departments to meet the needs of war. The majority of public health physicians, nurses, sanitarians, and other health department staff entered the military service. After the war ended there was some resurgence of interest in re-establishing local health units but financing and staff for them were very limited. In subsequent years, public health services became fragmented and dis-membered at the national, state, and local levels. One of the first major changes was made by the Congress. It removed responsibility for water pollution control, air pollution control, and environmental health programs from the USPHS and transferred them to a new environmental protection agency (E.P.A.). In this agency direction of programs was largely by politically oriented and politically appointed attorneys.

Emphasis changed from protecting public health using professionals trained in this field to control by legally oriented administrators.

In states and local communities responsibility for community mental health services, services for crippled children, school health, environmental health, public health laboratories, and, in some instances, vital statistics programs, were often transferred out of health departments. New programs such as those to control AIDS frequently were established in new agencies, disregarding the long record of major successes of health departments in combating and controlling serious communicable diseases. Such actions have resulted in the dismemberment of health departments in many communities. This sorry state of community public health services has been recognized for many years by governors' committees, study comissions, public health organizations, and most recently by a Presidential Commision on public health services. Unfortunately, conditions have only worsened.

As Director of Health and Mental Health in a moderate-sized county of California, as Director of Maternal and Child Health in the Oregon State Health Department, as Chief Deputy Director of Health in California for a number of years, and as State Health Officer and Director of the Oregon State Board of Health for fifteen years, I had the unique opportunity of witnessing the development of excellent public health programs, the radical changes in administration of these programs as they occurred, and the deterioration of these preventive services into the present chaotic state.

Currently numerous suggestions are being made for new types of health personnel in different agencies to meet public health needs, overlooking or forgetting the proven value of public health physicians, public health nurses and aides, health educators and other staff of health departments in case-finding, disease control, and community health education. These untoward developments are the basis for my concern. As I expressed them to members of my family, fellow physicians, public health personnel, teachers, friends, and others, I was encouraged to share, in writing, some of my many experiences, my observations on changes in the public health infrastructure, and my concerns. Equally important, to make suggestions on how to reach the excellent goals that have been established.

I have written in general terms to make the book more interesting not only to health personnel, but to students, the public, and to all who have an interest in the prevention of disease and the promotion of good health.

That is the "why?" of this book.

1. Evolvement of Health Departments

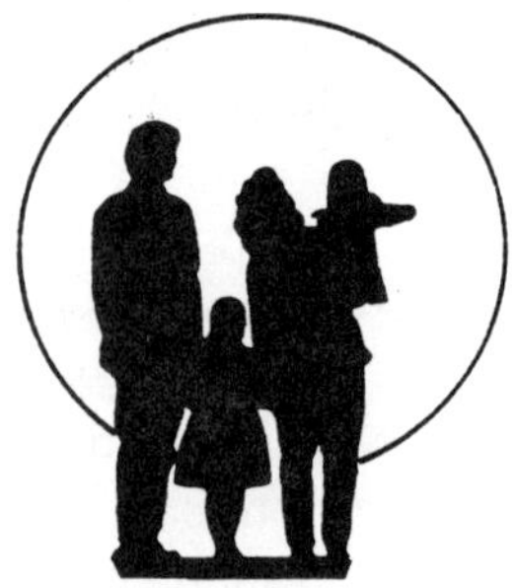

PUBLIC HEALTH CONDITIONS at the beginning of this century were substantially different from those of today. Communicable disease was rampant. Families were being decimated by smallpox, diphtheria, typhoid fever, malaria, scarlet fever, meningitis, tuberculosis, syphilis, and other diseases. Babies and their mothers were particularly susceptible to infections. Life expectancy at the turn of the century was about forty to forty-five years. Nearly half the babies died before the age of five years. Many succumbed in infancy. Many more died in early childhood, attacked by one or more of the infectious diseases, or due to malnutrition. Mothers often had many children, not only to insure the survival of a few, but because contraceptive methods were crude and often ineffective. In those children that survived, the incidence of blindness, deafness, paralysis, or other physical or mental disabilities was high. Bacteria had not been identified as the cause of many infections— and viruses had only recently been discovered. There were no antibiotics. U.S. Census data first collected in 1790 was far from accurate. Official records of births and deaths and of communicaable diseases were incomplete. In many areas of the country the only record of births and deaths was in a family bible.

The residents of Massachusetts deserve credit for recognizing the need for vital statistics and collecting them. In 1639 the Massachusetts Bay Colony began to require the reporting of births, deaths, and marriages. Prior to this time, the only public records were those in churches. It was recognized that these were generally incomplete and insufficient for legal purposes, inheritances, and evaluations of the populations. Assuring the collection of this vital data was a step in strengthening the populace's common bond, and in making their government responsible for protecting this essential information. The communication of ideas, subsequent adoption of them, and progress are often slow. It was not until 1799, some 160 years later, that the City of Boston recognized the need for an arm of the government to gather additional data on the residents health status, to analyze causes of death, and to take organized steps to protect the communities health that individuals could not take. To do this the city created the first health department in this country.

At this time there were few hospitals and those that did exist were more likely to be charnel houses (places to die) rather than facilities for recovery. There were no standards for them nor were they licensed. Some isolation hospitals (often called pest houses), were maintained for quarantine purposes. The practice of dentistry was largely that of extracting teeth.

Discoveries in the nineteenth century were to make dramatic changes in medical, dental, nursing, and hospital practices in this century. They would make possible the prevention of many communicable diseases as well as their control. To fully appreciate the dramatic changes that influenced the development of public health services let us consider some of these discoveries. Ignaz Semmelweiss, a Hungarian physician, introduced antisepsis* into lying-in wards with great success in the reduction of maternal deaths. Joseph Lister, a Scottish Physician, revolutionized surgery by introducing antisepsis in surgery in 1865. Florence Nightingale, during the Crimean war, demonstrated in the army hospital wards the value of nursing care and sanitation by keeping patients and the wards free of waste, and clean. She also assured the patients wholesome food and water.** Civilian hospitals soon adopted similar procedures. Between 1862 and 1890, she established an effective system of hospital schools for training nurses. Roentgen discovered the x-ray in 1895 and it was adapted to medical, dental and public health use in the early part of this century. In 1895 while in the Dutch east indies, Christian Eijkman discovered that polishings from rice would prevent beriberi. Extracts were called thiamine or vitamin B1. This was the first recognition of a specific cause of a vitamin deficiency disease. Although the value of citrus fruits in prevention of scurvy had been recognized earlier, it was not until this time, and largely through animal experimentation that lack of vitamin C was proven to be the cause of scurvy.

*The use of killing agents such as lysol and tincture of iodine to destroy bacteria and other microorganisms that can cause disease.

**TLC—tender loving care undoubtedly was a factor assisting her to success.

Soon a number of other vitamins essential for life and the prevention of disease were found. These discoveries and the discovery of hormones and other findings including the importance of trace elements such as iodine, fluoride, iron, and zinc, also made dramatic changes in nutritional science in the prevention and treatment of deficiency diseases.

In the latter part of the nineteenth century important developments had a major impact on the control of communicable diseases and improved sanitation.

The discoveries of Louis Pasteur, the great French scientist and a true humantitarian, were some of the most important in advancing public health. These included establishment of the germ theory in 1877 following his discovery of a bacillus causing the death of silkworms in France. Through exquisite epidemiology he demonstrated the natural history of anthrax and soon produced effective attenuated vaccines to prevent anthrax in cattle, and chicken cholera in fowl. On July 6, 1885, he successfully inoculated a boy who had been severely bitten by a rabid dog. Again he used an attenuated virus.*

Frederich Loffler's discovery in 1898 of the virus causing hoof and mouth disease in cattle and proving beyond a doubt that it was a virus, an infectious agent which had not been recognized before, was an important milestone. His earlier finding with Klebs in 1879 of the bacillus causing diphtheria which led to production of antitoxin (1892), and later to toxoid, and a skin test (Schick) for diphtheria was essential to a control program. Such discoveries and newer knowledge of the extent of the problems also made possible the prevention and control of many of the communicable and nutritional deficiency diseases and improvement of sanitation. It also made possible the assurance of safe water and milk supplies and radical changes in the concept and operation of hospitals.

Extensive knowledge about communicable disease existed. The problem was how to disseminate and apply this knowledge. A means for action had to be created. When causes of death were analyzed, and recorded from death certificates, the extent of communicable diseases became

*Edward Jenner had made a major contribution to immunization in 1796 when he refined and used cowpox secretions to vaccinate against smallpox.

apparent and resulted in an upsurge of interest in there control. As physicians reviewed these records they were alarmed with the number of deaths from yellow fever, smallpox, typhoid fever, diphtheria, scarlet fever, malaria, meningitis and other communicable disease. Leaders in medicine recognized that private physicians alone could not control the infectious diseases. They could not collect the necessary data. They had no authority to isolate communicable disease patients. They could not provide public health laboratory services, nor did they have the means of widely disseminating the newer knowledge.

Together with support of medical societies and public health associations, physicians provided the leadership which influenced state legislatures, city councils and Congress to establish boards of health and health departments.

Again Massachusetts led the way when the state legislature established the first of the nations state boards of health. The board was to serve the entire state. Concern and progress was not limited to Massachusetts. California established its state board of health in 1871. In the early 1900's many city and state boards of health and departments were established. By 1913 every state had a state board of health. The primary purpose of these boards was to control communicable disease. This was accomplished through collecting vital statistics and data on these diseases, quarantining or isolating individuals having them and instituting other essential measures to control the infections. In addition, water supplies and milk supplies were to be scrutinized for safety and sanitation was to be improved. Public health laboratories were established in these city and state health departments as a part of the communicable disease control program.

Along with these developments in cities and states, the federal government recognized that it had a responsibility for public health. The Congress had established the United States Marine Hospital Service (USMHS), in 1798. In 1879, responding to the same kind of interest being expressed in the states and cities, the Congress established a National Board of Health. This board was responsible directly to the President of the United States. Initially its role was to cooperate with the state and city boards of health, to collect data on communicable disease and sanitation, and to quarantine regions, ships, or ports as necessary. Recognizing duplications in responsibilities of the USMHS and the National Board of Health, the Congress, in August of 1882, limited the National Board to activities strictly for the control of yellow fever, cholera, and smallpox. The National Board members' terms of four years expired in March of 1883. At that time its responsibilities were transfered to the USMHS. With increasing interest in community health, Congress expanded this service in 1902 to a Public Health and Marine Hospital Service. In 1912 Congress designated it as The United States Public Health Service (USPHS). A Surgeon General for the USMHS had been appointed in 1870. Outstanding physician-surgeons were appointed to direct the federal, state, and city health departments. The selection of these directors was based on their professional abilites and interest in public health. Politics, as such, played no part in appointments. Tenure depended on performance. At that time it was said that responsibility for public health was being taken from the politicians and given to the well-qualified professionals! (Quite a contrast to current practices.)

EARLY LEADERSHIP

The first Surgeon General of the USMHS, Dr. John M. Woodworth was a dynamic leader. He visualized a National Health Department with broad public health responsibility rather than merely that of providing medical care for seamen. He was a tireless worker. Under his direction an effective national quarantine program was established. This was the first federal government action relating to quarantine in over 75 years. Dr. Woodworth emphasized the need for the supervision of ocean travel to assure good sanitation, for inspection of crews and passengers of ships for serious communicable diseases, detaining those found to be infected. He stressed the necessity for international cooperation. He was active in the planning and forming of the American Public Health Association, and converted the loosely connected, locally appointed physicians into a highly qualified team available for service in any part of the country, when needed to control communicable disease outbreaks. His untimely death in March of 1879 after nine years of service was followed by the appointment of Dr. John B. Hamilton, who was only thirty-two years of age at the time of his selection. He established goals for the Service and energetically pursued them. These included the development of an interstate quarantine system, in March of 1890, it was established by an act of Congress. The system was designed to prevent the transmission of infectious disease from one state to another. During Dr. Hamilton's tenure the Hygienic

Laboratory, (which later was a factor in the establishment of the National Institute of Health), was organized in 1887 at the Marine Hospital in New York city. Considerable assistance was given to the states in the investigation and control of epidemics, particularly yellow fever. After twelve years of service as Surgeon General, Dr, Hamilton resigned in 1891.

I dwell on the role of these early Surgeon Generals to illustrate the type of leadership that these men gave, their vital program accomplishments during these early developmental stages of the USPHS and to emphasize the benefits of continuity in leadership that instituted communicable disease control measures, and established important federal-state and international relationships. Dr. Walter Wynn was appointed as the third Surgeon General of the USMHS in 1891. During his twenty years of service major advances were made in reorganization of the USMHS and in improving national health. Among the many accomplishments during his tenure were extension of the quarantine system to U.S. territories; creation in 1902 by treaty with other nations, of the Pan-American Sanitary bureau, and of the International Office of Public Health in Paris; Congressional authorization and establishment of annual and special conferences of the Surgeon General with State and Territorial Health Authorities; Congressional authorization to license production of biologicals to be sold in interstate commerce; and the reorganization and expansion of the USMHS in 1902 into the U.S. Public Health and Marine Hospital Service.

In 1902 Surgeon General Wyman called the first Surgeon General's conference with the State and Territoral Health Officers. This was to be one of the many important annual meetings to discuss public health problems, establish plans to resolve them, and to exchange information on successes and failures in conducting programs.

In 1912, Surgeon General Rupert Blue was successful with the authorization from Congress in further recognizing and increasing the effectiveness of what was now the USPHS. Dr. Blue stressed improved sanitation particularly in rural areas. He promoted the establishment of local health departments. During the eight years that Dr. Blue served as Surgeon General of the USPHS, a nationwide program for control of venereal disease was inaugerated; a research laboratory to study stream pollution was established in Cincinnati, Ohio; a national leprosarium was authorized by Congress; and systematic programs were instituted to study and control malaria and trachoma. A more comprehensive national public health program was being developed.

The USPHS had been fortunate in having such well qualified and truly outstanding leaders as Surgeon Generals. Until recent years partisan politics played little part in their appointments. They were career public health physicians selected from the USPHS Corps, based on their training, experience, and knowledge of public health. They had had wide experience in the field investigations and control of communicable disease outbreaks, they had worked with state and local health departments, and they had increasingly responsible administrative experience.

During these years the public, as reflected by the legislative actions of Congress and state legislatures, became more aware of the importance of public health and the necessity for the government to protect it. A significant change reflecting this awareness in Congress was the transfer in 1939 of the USPHS from the jurisdiction of the U.S. Treasury Department to the Federal Security Agency.

Under the guidance of Surgeon Generals Hugh Smith Cummings, and Thomas Parran, the National Institute of Health and the present Clinical Center were established. Dr. Lewis R. Thompson, who became the first Director of the combined division Scienfific Research and National Institute of Health in 1937, deserves real recognition for his part in the development of the present Clinical Centers. On direction from Surgeon General Cummings, Dr. Thompson met with Mr. and Mrs. Luke Wilson and fostered their great interest in medical research. They were so impressed that they made an initial gift to the USPHS in 1935, of forty-five acres of valuable land adjacent to Bethesda, Maryland. In 1937, although Mr. Luke had passed away, his wife, her son and his wife, gave another forty-five acres and the cottages on them, to the Service. It was on this land that the world renowned Clinical Center was built. The Congress appropriated one hundred million dollars in 1935, for buildings and new institutes. This and additional appropriations for buildings, staff, equipment, research, and for grants to other institutions for research have made possible the tremendous medical research program as it now exists—the finest in the world.

The other unit of the USPHS is the Communicable Disease Center (CDC), based in Atlanta, Georgia. It was established under Surgeon General Parran's direction in 1940. This center with its staff of eminent epidemiologists, laboratory, and other professional personnel, cooperates with state and local health departments in the study, prevention, and control of communicable disease. The CDC has operational units in environmental health,

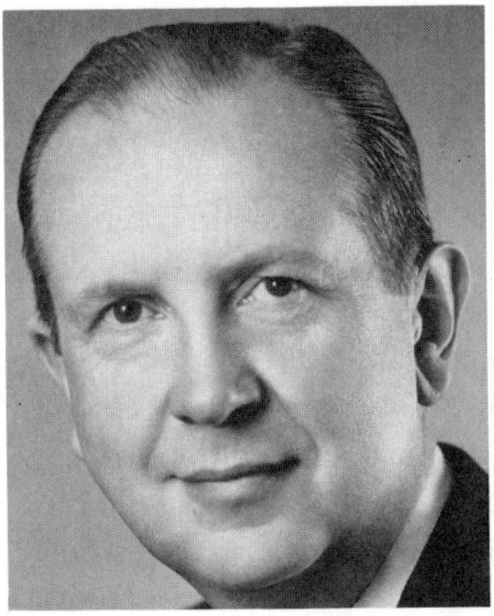

Surgeon General Leonard A. Scheele

health education, and it has a National Institute for Occupational Safety and Health.

The record of accomplishment of both of these units, and of the USPHS as a whole is a tribute to the Directors who have been able to develop programs with the full support of Congress, the states and many professional and non-professional organizations as well as private citizens interested in public health.

I would be remiss in this brief review if I did not mention the contributions of Surgeon General Leonard A. Scheele★ to the National Institutes. Under his direction the National Institutes of Heart, Dental Research, Arthritis, and Metabolic Diseases, and the Institutes of Neurological Diseases and Blindness were added. The National "Institute" of Health became the National "Institutes" of Health in 1948. The National Water Pollution Control Program and the Environmental Health Center iin Cincinnati, Ohio, were also established under Dr. Scheele's direction. Of even greater significance was the recognition of the need for cooperation and the establishment of a partnership between the federal government and the states in protecting the nation's health. The need for funds and the most effective means of expending them were key elements in the discussion.

Paralleling these federal activities were developments at the state level. Outstanding physicians were appointed by state boards of health as State Health Officers, to develop and direct state health department programs. As in the federal government, appointments were based on training and experience, not on political affiliation. As Governor E. G. (Pat) Brown of California told me in the early sixties, "Membership in a particular political party should not influence appointments to public health positions".

I had the privilege of serving as one of the three United States delegates to the World Health Assembly in Geneva, Switzerland, in 1954, and during the three weeks that we were there I became well-acquainted with, and came to respect Dr. Scheele for his ability and his affability. He was an effective delegate.

Outstanding leaders such as Dr. Samuel J. Crumbine, State Health Officer of Kansas, Dr. John H. Hurty, State Health Officer of Indiana, and many others had remarkable public health leadership records. Dr. Crumbine is remembered for his successful campaigns in combating typhoid fever and other communicable diseases, in controlling houseflies and in abolishing the common drinking cup and towel. Dr. Hurty was known for his success in fighting tuberculosis, venereal disease and acute infectious disease. Dr. Charles V. Chapin of Rhode Island probably holds the all-time record for length of service, forty-eight years (from 1884 through 1932). Joseph N. McCormick, M.D., and Arthur T. McCormick, M.D., father and son, served Kentucky as State Health Officers for fifty-nine years! Notable accomplishments were made possible by continuity in office, as well as support from an appreciative public.

PLAN FOR LOCAL HEALTH UNITES FOR THE NATION

I have considered the early development of city boards of health and city health departments as pioneered by Boston, Philadelphia, and Baltimore. Many cities throughout the nation also recognized the need for health departments and established them. The groundswell of action by physicians, medical societies, public health organizations, and the general public to motivate federal, state, and city governmental action to protect the public health did not extend to counties until 1911. A typhoid outbreak in Yakima county, Washington, stimulated the formation of one of the first county health departments in the United States at that time. Guilford County, North Carolina, also established a county health department in that year. Jefferson County, Virginia, may have had a health department as early as 1908. In any event, the value of these departments was soon recognized in many areas of the country. By 1921, one hundred eighty-six county health departments had been established in twenty-three states.

In many areas not served by full-time county health departments, schools employed school nurses, counties employed public health nurses, and most counties were required by state laws to employ as a minimum, a physician-surgeon as a part-time health officer. Many county public health associations, affiliates of state and national tuberculosis associations were organized in the mid and late thirties. With enthusiastic and effective support of the latter, often including financial support, and through cooperation of schools and counties many more full-time county health departments were created.

The earlier establishment of the Childrens bureau (CB), in the Department of Labor in 1912, to promote public health services for mothers and children, and enactment of the Shepard-Towner Act in 1921, the first major grant-in-aid program for health, indirectly aided in promoting the formation of county health departments. One of the most significant advances came in 1935 with the enactment of the Social Security Act. Federal Funds became available both through the USPHS and the CB for assisting states, counties, and health districts in the establishment and maintainance of adequate health services, including the training of personnel for state and local health work. This action assured the possibility of good community health service for everyone. With this new incentive additional county health departments were established. Large numbers of physicians, public health nurses, sanitarians, statisticians, sanitary engineers, dentists, and health educators entered the field of public health. Many received stipends for advanced training in public health, usually leading to a master's degree for most, a doctorate degree in public health for others. This special training included studies in epidemiology; communicable disease control; public health administration; collection and analysis of vital statistics; preventive health services including programs for mothers and children; sanitary science; occupational health; public health and laboratory techniques; nutrition; and health education.

The promotional work of many organizations and the interest of the public in health was bringing results. As I state in another chapter, by 1941 about two thirds of the population of the country was being served by full-time local health departments, although in many instances these departments were skeletal. Full-timc was defined as having a full-time physician, preferably trained in public health, as director, and additional full-time staff including public health nurses, sanitarians and essential clerical personnel.

During this important period of major development of local health services (1910-1941), the support of leaders in Congress, federal, state and local government, officials, state boards of health, organizations such as the American Public Health Association (APHA), AMA, National Tuberculosis Association (NTA), Rockefeller Foundation and the dedicated work of individuals brought real results. The contributions of men such as Dr. Leslie L. Lumsden, (USPHS), DRS. Haven Emerson and Carl Buck (APHA), and Dr. John A. Ferrell (Rockefeller Foundation), and local leaders were incalculably important in reaching the goal of "Local Health Units (and services) for the Nation."

Funds appropriated by Congress for public health included grants for tuberculosis control, venereal disease control, maternal and child health, and for "General Health." The latter were intended to help states establish local health departments. Based on the need for training of public health personnel, and as a result of urging by the APHA, State and Terrritorial Health Officers, and other organizations, Congress appropriated additional monies specifically for public health training. Funds were included to support Schools of Public Health.

Public Health experienced momentous changes during the years between 1937 and 1941. With the availability of federal matching funds, state and local governments, many for the first time, appropriated funds to establish local health departments and to expand others. A large number of physicians, nurses, and others interested in prevention were atttracted to careers in public health. As mentioned earlier, many received or obtained a year or more of special training in the field. Stipends of federal funds, granted by the states, assisted many students in getting this additional education.

Dr, Haven Emerson, a renowned public health physican, under the auspices of the APHA, made a study of the public health needs of the country and developed a plan providing for county, district, and city health departments to serve the entire United States. This "plan" was generally supported by most health organizations, national, state, and local. Some revisions were indicated, but as a whole, it was considered to be an excellent plan that would markedly improve the public health if it was implemented.

The Plan envisaged local Health Units serving geographical areas with 40,000 or more population. Each Unit or Health Department would be directed by a full-time physician trained in public health and administration. Staff would include one public health nurse or aide for each 5,000-8,000 persons in the area, and one sanitarian, and health educator for each 40,000-50,000 residents. Likewise to be included were a public health laboratory either in the department or readily available; adequate clerical staff, and consultating services of sanitary engineers, public health dentists, nutritionists, statisticians, and other public health specialists (usually provided by the state.) In the Plan the entire United States was divided into logical geographical areas which would encompass a population of

40,000 or more. Adequate office and clinic space would be available in one or more centers in the area served. (Necessary office and clinic furniture, equipment, and supplies would be provided. Transportation for the staff would be arranged.)

This staff, working along side the community's physicians, dentists, hospitals (local or in an adjacent area), schools, other health personnel, and organizations interested in community health, would determine what the major health problems were, what resources were available to resolve them, and initiate programs towards this end.

Financial support would be from federal USPHS and CB Grants, (dispersed by the states); state funds as available; and local government, volunteer organizations, and private funds.

The program would include collection and analysis of vital statistics (birth, death, marriage, in some instances divorce data), collection of records on incidence of communicable disease (CD), and analysis of them, prevention and control of CDs, maintainance of a hygenic laboratory to aid in this control, provision of preventive health services for mothers, infants, and children, protection of water, milk, and food supplies, vector control (mosquitos, rodents, flies, etc.), diagnosis and treatment of persons with sexually transmitted diseases (STDs), and health education. Particular emphasis would be placed on public health nursing visits to homes to counsel with and motivate pregnant women to get pre-natal care early in their pregnancy, to cooperate with the woman's own physician in assuring continued pre-natal, delivery and post-partum care. These public health nurses (and aides) would likewise visit women, children, and others in the home to ensure immunizations and preventive health care of babies, pre-school, (and school) children. They would follow cases of tuberculosis, other infectious diseases, and individuals found in screening programs. They would uncover contacts of CD, and STD cases and check on them to assure diagnosis and treatment of those infected.

Well-baby, pre-school, and school health clinics would be conducted for immunizations, vision and hearing screenings, and to find children in need of medical care. Those children who had personal physicians would be referred to them. Those who did not would be assisted in selecting a physician or clinic for care. Community health education programs would be carried on by the health educator and by all members of the staff as they provided services. Periodic evaluation of progress being made with changes in the program as indicated was envisioned.

This is only a brief summary of activities planned for "Local Health Units for the Nation." If the plan was fully implemented, it would provide a real bulwark of defense against the spread of C.D. and S.T.D. It would assure that most women would receive pre-natal and obstetrical care, that infants, pre-school, and school children were immunized early, and that most of those who had physical or mental disabilities would be found and receive good medical and dental care. Water, milk, and food supplies would be well supervised and safe. Communities would receive sound health education through co-operation with schools, T.V., radio, and news media, and voluntary health organizations. Those who needed health information would have opportunities for individual face-to-face, counselling, questioning, and discussion. A major advantage of the Plan would be that such services would be well co-ordinated and a true liaison developed between the public health nurses (PHN aides) and the families or individuals whom they served. This would assure a level of good "primary prevention" health care that would be very difficult to achieve in any other way!*

As health departments were established and strengthened they were better able to evaluate community health problems, to work with physicians, dentists, school personnel, and the citizenry in resolving them. They were able to present to Congress, to state legislatures, and to local government, convincing data on the need for and the value of health department services. Statistics and records showed the United States had one of the highest infant and maternal mortality rates of any industrialized country in the world, and that only a small percentage of infants and children were adequately immunized, that relatively few expectant mothers were receiving adequate pre-natal care, and that the large majority of children were not not receiving preventive health services. Thousands of infants were dying from whooping cough, small pox, diphtheria, scarlet fever, polio, typhoid fever, and other acute C.D.s. Tuberculosis and syphilis were rampant. The latter resulted in 10% of the patients in mental institutions being there due to paresis (syphilis of the brain). In the few areas with established health departments, records showed a marked contrast in results from attacking these problems.

By 1941, about two-thirds of the country was served by local health departments. It seemed that soon, the greater part of the nation would thus be served. This did not happen. World War II interrupted and disrupted local health services that had been established. Much of the financial

*More detail on these and other activities of health departments will be discussed in later chapters.

support for local health services, and particularly for prevention, was redirected to medical care and war-related services. In addition, civilian hospitals, medical clinics, and health departments lost much of their staff to military services. The need for physicians and nurses suddenly increased radically. Medical schools that had received some federal support for expansion before World War II, now received large grants to train many new doctors. The size of classes was increased and accelerated schedules of training reduced the length of training from four years to three, by extending classes from nine months to twelve.

Staffs of state and local health departments were decimated during the war, due to military needs. To help fill a part of this gap, particularly the loss of public health physicians, the USPHS recruited physicians, commissioned them as PHS Officers and assigned them to fill key positions in state and local health departments. Without this assistance, most health departments and the services which they provided would have vanished.

The Public Health Service followed a policy in recruitment and assignment of personnel which probably was a result of war psychology and a belief that there should be a personal sacrifice on the part of the physicians. Public health physcians, well acquainted with the health problems, resources, and programs in the area they served, when recruited, were removed from their positions and transferred to another geographical area, often across the continent. In the new location, the physician, of necessity, had to acquaint himself or herself with a completly different situation, which frequently took months. This was an inefficient way to utilize scarce personnel.

The War did result in advances in knowledge on how to control many communicable diseases, in disaster planning and care, and in rehabilitation (in addition to advances in medicine, orthopedics, and surgery). Although Health Departments are only tangentially involved in rehabilitation of cases previously considered to be "hopeless"; this dramatic change is worthy of illustration.

A relatively young attorney had been in an automobile accident and had suffered a broken neck with spinal cord injury resulting in quadriplegia (paralysis of both legs, both arms, and the body). The young man had resigned himself to spending the rest of his life in a nursing home. Dr. Howard Rusk, a pioneer in the field of rehabilitation, heard of the young man and traveled many miles to visit him. Dr. Rusk explained and offered the help that he was giving to others suffering similar conditions. This individual, confined in a nursing home, initially was not impressed and refused Dr. Rusk's offer. Dr. Rusk, somewhat in disgust and in a final effort, told the man that he thought an attorney practiced law utilizing his brain, eyes, ears, and mouth, not his arms and legs! Spurred by this challenge, the patient later accepted admission to Dr. Rusk's rehabilitation center, in New York City, and after several months of rehabilitation therapy and training in use of a special motorized wheelchair, he was rehabilitated. Later he was offered a position writing legal contracts for a major corporation and proved to be one of the best lawyers they had ever had. Similar cases, returning handicapped persons, stroke patients, and others to productive life illustrated the new successes in rehabilitation.

I have referred to the stagnation of the program to establish full-time health services for the entire nation, as the result of loss of personnel and funds during the World War II years. Soon thereafter efforts were made to re-vitalize the Plan. Personnel were recruited to fill postions vacated during the war. Many physicians, nurses, sanitary engineers, sanitarians, health educators, and other types of health department staff received public health training.

This was due, not only to federal financial support for schools of public Health, but also to the interest in public health stimulated by experience in the war, and as a result of witnessing the success of public health programs. War veterans took advantage of funds available for training in public health. I have talked with many young physicians and medical corpsmen who served in World War II (and others who served in Korea and Vietnam) who were greatly impressed by the effectiveness of public health measures in the control of communicable disease. They also appreciated the value of health education, good sanitation, and health maintenance services for the military. Many of these physicians, medical corpsmen, and nurses, too, entered the public health field.

Between 1945 and 1960 much progress was made in restoring and providing good health department services. A number of new programs were established and others expanded by states and local government. These programs included hospital construction; mental health; dental health; services for crippled children; "venereal" (S.T.D.) disease, tuberculosis, and chronic disease control; occupational health; migrant health; and air pollution control. Others were school health programs; services for mothers, infant and pre-school children; screening programs for adults, and health programs for senior citizens. Licensing of hospitals, nursing homes, and related facilities as well as the licensing of restaurants were instituted. General sanitation was improved. Milk and water supplies were closely guarded. Water pollution and radiation control, as well as home and motor vehicle safety programs were established or expanded.

For many reason, however, the earlier impetus to provide local public health services for every citizen, urban and rural, was never fully regained. Funds previously made available by the Congress for establishment and expansion of Health Departments were now limited.

Although there are approximately 3,000 local health departments in the United States today, about two-thirds are small and most are extremely understaffed. Arkansas, Deleware, Rhode Island, and Vermont do not have local health departments. California did achieve a goal of making local public health services available to all its residents. Legislation was enacted providing state funds to assist all counties in the state in establishing and maintaining such services. In smaller counties where it was not practical to establish full-time health departments, the state provided funds and consultation for locally employed public health nurses, sanitarians, and clerical personnel. Most states were never able to, or chose not to, establish such service or financial assistance for sparsely settled areas. One-third of the states elected to provide community health services utilizing state-employed, rather than locally-employed staff. The services generally were the basic ones as previously discussed: (1) maintain vital records and records of communicable disease, (2) control communicable disease, (3) maintain public health laboratory service, (4) develop preventive health services for mothers and children, (5) protect water, milk, and food supplies and maintain other essential sanitation services, and (6) conduct health education programs to promote better health practices. Major emphasis was on prevention. Treatment for sexually transmitted disease (STD) was usually provided to prevent the spread of infections. Individuals suffering from tuberculosis who could not afford treatment generally received it. Mental health and crippled children's services were added later.

FRAGMENTATION AND DE-PROFESSIONALIZATION

Several factors detailed in the chapter "Politics in Health," began to change the character of health agencies and the way in which services were provided. This occurred at all levels of government. The Congress, probably responding to special health interests, began the process of fragmentation by making funds for preventive health services available to other agencies as well as health departments. Responsibility for Administration of crippled children;s services, mental health, hospital construction, hospital planning, occupational health, environmental health, and many other public health services was given to seperate agencies in many states. This fragmentation became most apparent beginning in the sixties.

In 1962, studies revealed that fourteen special kinds of health services were being provided to half a milllion children in California. The authors concluded that health care provided with tax funds was a "confusing, fragmented, jumble" involving many agencies. "Care was seldom comprehensive or coordinated." Another sudy likewise concluded that federal, state, and local governments developed a multitude of largely unrelated health services to meet special needs. These services were offered in a "patchwork of piecemeal and overlapping programs." Toward the end of the century, the situation grew worse. One study revealed more than forty seperate health programs. The federal block grant approach was an attempt to resolve some of the fragmentation, but unfortunalty, much of the damage had been done.

"In the interest of centralizing authority and coordination", reorganization took place at national, state, and local levels. Nationally the Department of Health, Education and Welfare, which succeeded the Federal Security Agency, was divided. A new Department of Education was created. An effort to get a separate Department of Health was never successful. Later, the Department of Health and Welfare was re-named the Department of Health and Human Resources. The status of the Surgeon General of th USPHS was weakened by establishing supervisory positions filled by political appointees. The responsibilities for water pollution control, air pollution control, and other environmental health services were removed from the USPHS and given to a new agency, the Environmental Protection Agency.

In most states, boards of health , members of which were outstanding, well-qualified persons serving without pay, were abolished. Many of these boards had advised and helped to guide successful public health programs for over a century. Apparently this record of service was considered to be irrelevant. The reason usually given for abolishing them was to make direction of health services more responsible to the governor. State health departments and directors of them were subordinated in the new state organizations and in many instances similar dismantling occured in the counties. Qualifications for directors were revised or minimized to permit appointments based on political affiliations and support, rather than on professional training and experience in the field of public health.

By 1985, nine state health departments had non-physicians as directors. Questions began to arise as to the ability of non-physicians to handle public health emergencies. To illustrate, in 1985 a serious outbreak of salmonella occurred in the Chicago area. People questioned the non-physician state director's decision to delay action to control the outbreak while he vacationed for two weeks. The resulting public outcry forced the Governor to fire the director. He then appointed an attorney to the position but again the public opposed the appointment, and shortly the Governor replaced the attorney with a qualified, well-trained public health physician.

Similar de-professionaliztion occurred in other departments. Morale as well as programs suffered in many such cases. A classic example of using political supporters in place of qualified and well-trained, experienced professionals, as reported in the news media, was the decision by the then-Governor of California, Jerry Brown, to disregard the advice of professional experts in agriculture to take immediate action when a Mediterranean fruit fly infestation was discovered. It was reported that political appointees without any background in agriculture and contrary to the advice of the technical staff, advised the Governor not to institute a control program immediatly because of the likelihood of adverse publicity. There was a chance the problem would go away. The Governor accepted the latter advice. Delay in control permitted the spread of the "Med Fly" and the following year a much more extensive control program, costing millions of dollars, was required. Again, according to the press, the delay cost the people of California hundreds of millions of dollars as a result of the embargoes on California fruit by other states and foreign countries, fruit losses, and the greatly increased cost of spray eradication programs.

Other changes were being made in public health. Health planning was fragmented. One third of the programs were administered by new agencies. Regions established for planning often were unrealistic, impractical, and required repeated changes. Waste and fraud were reported in some of these agencies. Congress finally withdrew all funds for the program.

Similar changes occurred in the counties. In many areas, environmental health and santitation were taken out of county health departments and placed in new seperate departments. Mental health, school health, crippled children services, licensing of health facilities, public health laboratories, vital statistics, and health education were often assigned to agencies other than health departments. In many local departments, public health physicians were replaced as directors by non-physicians. The reasons for this change most frequently given were that there were a shortage of such physicians, that others could administer public health programs equally well, or better, that salary savings could be made, and that it was a waste of physicians' time to involve them in administration. It was said that physicians could be called in when medical advice was required. The effect on program quality, morale, and costs of such measures taken in the interest of economy needs to be ascertained. Were these assumptions correct? Have health services improved or worsened? Are costs less or greater?

Those who question qualified public health physician direction of health departments should consider the importance of planning and implementing public health programs as a part of total health care. Can an individual, not medically trained, recognize the potentials of early signs of communicable disease outbreaks, or other threats to the community's health, as well as a physician with specialized training in public health and administration? Can non-physicians be as effective in working with physicians if they are not a part of the medical community? Are their pronouncements on public health accepted by the public as well as those of a physician? Would Surgeon General C. Everett Koop's statements on AIDS, smoking, and "driving while under the influence" have been as effective if he had not been recognized as a well-qualified physician?

In addition to changes in qualifications of directors of public health departments, other changes have occurred. State and local health agencies have been increasingly involved in medical care, with a corresponding dilution of preventive health services. Fees are now being charged, or nominal fees increased for many services, including sanitary inspections, laboratory services, clinical services, copies of and searches for vital records and for some health education materials. The basic concept of providing preventive health services and control measures for communicable diseases as a tax supported service in the interest of the total population is being changed. Now, preventive health and medical care services are being provided by the government, often in competition with private facilities and, in some instances, charging fees greater than those of non-governmental providers.

Justification for this is that services would not otherwise be available and that people should pay for care based on their ability to pay.

Some important questions need to be answered. How are these changes affecting public health and at what cost? Are the multiple agencies doing well-coordinated health planning? Are services for individuals and families adequate? Are they complete and well-coordinated, or are they fragmented and superficial? Are the public health problems of the communities being adequately diagnosed and treated?

In many instances these consolidations, reorganizations, fragmentations, dispersions of responsibility for health services, de-professionalization, and greater political dictation have led to chaos, poor morale, resignations, and early retirement of well-qualified professional staff. Often they have discouraged young people from entering the field of public health. Not only are many health departments being dissected, but very few new ones are being established. Many have been abolished. Over one fourth of our nation's population is as of yet not served by any kind of local health department. Why? Is there no longer a need for nationwide community, preventive, public health services? What is the current status of public health?

2. Crisis in Public Health

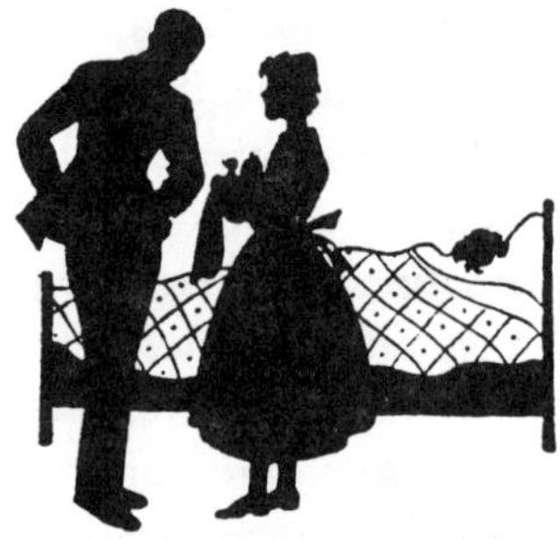

MOST AUTHORITIES AGREE that there is a crisis in public health today. What is its extent, and what brought it about? The American Public Health Association devoted an entire annual meeting to consideration of the crisis. A national commission, after much study, concluded that we are facing a real crisis. Many state studies have revealed that public health services are fragmented, are not coordinated, and that there is great confusion as to responsibilities, and as to the significance of this problem.

The United States is now confronted with an epidemic—some consider it a pandemic—of AIDS. In the past, we have expected health departments to institute measures to control such epidemics. Health Education is important, but even more vital is the need to identify individuals harboring the HIV (AIDS virus), and to take measures to prevent its spread. To do this requires mass screening, particularly of persons at special risk such as drug abusers. Someone needs to interpret the meaning of a positive laboratory test for the HIV, to allay unnecessary fears until the results of the initial test can be confirmed. They need to counsel with those actually infected with the virus. It is vital that they convince the latter of the importance of revealing their contacts. The necessity of finding those contacts, explaining the possibility of infection, the character of infection, and the importance of protecting others, is obvious. But who will do this?

Private physicians can handle some of the task. They can treat patients with Aids Related Complex (ARC), with AIDS, or those initially infected with the HIV, who come to their offices. Few, if any, however, are prepared, nor do they have the necessary staff to do the epidemiology, the "shoe leather" job to learn of, and to follow up on, contacts. But if the private physicians cannot do this, again, who will?

In the past we have expected Health Departments to manage this type of consultation and follow-up. We have depended on them to protect our communities' health, to guard against and to limit the spread of epidemics, to come to our aid in natural disasters, to maintain safe milk, water, and food supplies, to assure cleanliness in restaurants and health facilities, and to provide preventive health services essential to the promotion and preservation of good community health.

Now, adequately staffed health departments are not available to a large segment of our population and the State Boards of Health that had served the people so well, many for over one hundred years, have been abolished. These boards were responsive to the people. They employed well-qualified staffs and maintained high standards of performance. They held public hearings to assure that all concerned parties might be heard on proposed regulations before they were adopted. They were made up of responsible health and business leaders who volunteered their services in the interest of the public. By eliminating them, authority was centralized in the governors. Where education and experience requirements for Directors of state and local health departments were eliminated the door was opened often to appoint poorly qualified political supporters. In many places Health Departments, as such, were eliminated and consolidated into new super agencies. Many are so inadequately staffed that they cannot carry out their responsibilities effectively.

As I have explained, responsibilities have been so fragmented that a well-directed and coordinated service seems to be an impossibility. Planning for community health facilities was taken out of state health departments in many areas. The results were so disastrous* that the Congress in 1986, abolished the program. We have discussed the removal of responsibility for environmental health, mental health, occupational health, crippled children's services programs, radiation control, and even maintenance of vital health records from Health Departments and how they were assigned to other agencies.

The leadership of career public health physicians, many of whom had served their communities for many years, even decades, who were respected and who were relatively free of political interference, has now been lost in many states. According to a recent report of the AMA (American Medical Association) on residencies for advanced specialized training, there were

*As mentioned earlier.

only thirty-two physicians in training for positions in public health in the entire United States. Hundreds are needed. Even more disturbing is the fact that even fewer and fewer physicians are electing to seek careers in public health. Why? there certainly is a growing need for physicians specializing in public health. Some of these needs are emphasized by looking at what is happening to the public health.

By the eighties, tuberculosis, syphilis, whooping cough, measles, german measles, and other communicable diseases, which had been under control, began to increase. Half of the nation's children had not been immunized. In 1990 California declared a state-wide epidemic of measles! AIDS had appeared and was spreading, uncontrolled. Health departments were being further fragmented. Few, if any, new preventive health services were being proposed. To illustrate, osteoporosis, which causes hip or other fractures in twenty percent of women over age fifty, and similar public health problems, were being neglected. Although Operation Headstart served about half of three and four year olds, millions of children still were entering school with previously undetected vision, hearing, speech, other physical, and developmental defects. Many pregnant girls and women were not getting adequate pre-natal care.

The inadequacy of health departments to cope with health threatening emergenicies was well-illustrated in the Three Mile Island Nuclear Reactor Disaster in Pennsylvania. One of the first agencies to be called on for help was the State Health Department. A new well-qualified director learned that the department not only did not have anyone on its staff trained in nuclear radiation but it did not even have a library or a book on the subject!*

NECESSARY ACTIONS

What public health services should be available to achieve good community health? Every known case of tuberculosis, STD's, and patients with other infectious diseases should be assured of treatment and monitored, contacts determined, and follow-up, to limit spread, instituted. Surveilance for influenza and unusual communicable disease should be maintained. Expectant mothers not receiving care should be located, essential pre-natal care arranged for early in the pregnancy, and in cooperation with the

*We will discuss this in more detail later.

patient's physician, plans should be made for delivery. Public health nurses (PHN's), under the direction of the physician, should follow the mother and newborn baby with visits in the home to assure good health care for them. Infant and pre-school health clinics should be available for every child who otherwise would not receive this care. All infants and pre-school children should have protective immunizations. Although much valuable health education is incorporated in the PHN home visits and in the clinics, there should be a sufficient number of health educators, working with the schools and private agencies to organize and carry on effective community health education programs.

In cooperation with the schools, health departments should provide follow-up in the homes of children found through health screening examinations to be in need of medical care. Notices sent home with the child too often are ineffective. The need for immunizations should be explained in home and clinic visits and arrangements made for the immunizations as indicated.

In adults, in cooperation with the voluntary health agencies, health departments should provide follow-up on individuals found in health screening programs, on those who possibly have cancer, heart problems, high blood pressure, diabetes, cataracts, glaucoma, other eye pathology, or abnormal blood findings. Simply identifying persons who might have such conditions is of little value unless followed up.

Through good liaison with private physicians and hospitals accurate and complete records of births, deaths, and communicable diseases should be maintained. Based on analysis of these, and other pertinent information, programs to attack special problems and to improve community health should be planned. The need for hospitals, nursing homes, and other facilities should be studied and plans developed to assure comprehensive service without the waste of duplication, recognizing that irrespective of the source of funding construction, a major portion of the care in most facilities is financed by the government.

Assurance of safe water, milk, and food supplies should be achieved through constant monitoring. This should also apply to disposal of solid and toxic wastes.

Restaurants, swimming pools, hospitals, nursing homes, rest homes, hotels, motels, industrial plants, and other facilities should be inspected to assure that health standards are being met.

In cooperation with other community agencies plans should be made for natural disasters with realistic exercises to assure that medical supplies are available, that hospitals and physicians, nurses, pharmacists, ambulance companies, are well organized to provide immediate triage (sorting of patients for types of care), emergency treatment, transportatiion, and hospital, or field hospital care as needed.

Various types of preventive mental, dental, and health services should be provided. The developmentally retarded should not be overlooked.*

Additional services to protect the community's health, depending on the variable needs of the community, should be developed as the need for them becomes apparent. The services that I have outlined are somewhat ideal, but they are not unrealistic. Achieving them for our entire nation was the major goal in the plan for Local Helath Units For The Nation. Lack of them largely accounts for our crisis in public health today. The threatening spread of the AIDS virus is merely one illustration of the deficiency in our protective health network.

The American Medical Association recognized the need for better health planning and utilization of our resources. In 1982 it developed a project, "Health Policy Agenda for the American People". Almost two hundred public and private organizations were involved in this planning. Principles were developed and published. Task forces worked in six areas: Medical Science and Research; Education for Health Professionals; Health Manpower and Facilities; Delivery Mechanisms and Processes; Evaluation, Assessment and Control; and Payment for service. The major considerations involved medical care. This was highly commendable and greatly needed but where was the task force on preventive community health? Only four of some one hundred fifty-nine stated principles that were published relate specifically to public health and disease prevention! Others related to them tangentially. This is only one illustration of our neglect of the deteriorating preventive community health services as we concentrate on the more dramatic and important problems of providing curative medicine and surgery!

As mentioned, the American Public Health Association recently expressed its concern over what is happening to preventive health services. The theme of the meeting was, "Local Health Services: Crisis on the Front Line". Those professionals actually engaged in providing community health

*We will discuss such services in detail later.

services are in a position to recognize the undermining of our public health infrastructure. They see the dangers inherent in neglecting our preventive community health services. A national commission recently came to similar conclusions.*

Many excellent news stories have been written about the breakdowns that have occurred in our protective health systems. One series that was recognized as outstanding, and that won a national award, was written by Bruce Orwall, a journalist in Everett, Washington. On investigation of the local health department, he documented the fact that the department was underfunded, understaffed, and thus was failing to protect the public. The department was unable to make the necessary inspections of restaurants and food handling establishments. It was not maintaining standards or enforcing the legal requirements because of the inadequate numbers of staff. Orwall pointed out that deficiencies in protective health services were not peculiar to Snohomish County with "public health buried by bureaucracy" and no overall policy for public health issues.

Other coverage by the media has occurred, particularly when inadequacies of public health service become apparent, usually in emergency situations. There has been national recognition of malfeasance in office in the Environmental Protection Agency, of failure to enforce toxic waste disposal laws, and of failures in health reorganizations in Pennsylvania, California, Florida, and other states. Some changes have been made as a result of such publicity but these stories generally focus on the "tip of the iceberg", and fail to recognize the greater problem of national inadequacy of community public health services.

These are some of the aspects of the crisis in public health. Would there be such a crisis if the nation had adequate local health department service—if the "Plan" had been implemented?

WHY HAS THE "PLAN" FLOUNDERED?

What brought about this deterioration and failure to implement the plan to provide preventive community health services for everyone? Were health departments ineffective in combatting disease and in promoting better public health through community public health measures? Did the leadership

* In 1990, the A.M.A. recognized the dire need for Health departments and re-affirmed its support for "Local Health Units for the Nation."

of health departments fail? Were important public health problems overlooked? Did special interest groups envision advantages in seperate departments? Were the original goals of prevention overshadowed by involvement in medical care? Did politics account for failure to implement the plan? Was greater political control of health departments which resulted in reorganization, introduction of the spoils system and deprofessionalization in the best interests of the public? Did it result in better public health services?

Was it one of these or perhaps a combination of all of them that led to the collapse of the plans for "Local Health Units for the Nation" and "Model Standards for Community Preventive Health Services"?

One of the first and a vital question in determining the cause is whether health departments have functioned efficiently, and as expected, in controlling communicable disease, providing preventive community health services and in improving water, milk, and food supplies as well as general sanitation.

3. Records of Successes of Health Departments Combatting Communicable Disease

EARLY SCOURGES

One of the first challenges to health departments was the control of epidemics and communicable disease. Typhoid fever, diphtheria, smallpox, and yellow fever, were some of the early killers that destroyed families and struck fear in the population. Cholera and bubonic plague were constant threats.

CONTROL OF TYPHOID FEVER

Typhoid fever was one of the worst and most subtle of these diseases. It ravaged not only many parts of the United States, but many areas of the world between 1880 and 1900. Water supplies, milk, shellfish, and other foods were often contaminated with the typhoid bacteria. Raw sewage frequently containing typhoid organisms, poured into creeks, lakes, rivers, and ocean bays. Outhouses, "Chick Sales", or privies with shallow pits commonly were not merely the sources of pollution to nearby wells, but were also open to a profusion of houseflies that carried bacteria to food in kitchens and dining rooms. Typhoid carriers, although they were not yet known as such, helped to proliferate the disease.

As water supplies were chlorinated, typhoid patients and carriers quarantined, and public education programs carried on to explain how typhoid was spread, the incidence of disease declined. Campaigns were conducted to stop the use of common drinking cups, to protect wells, and to take other measures to protect individuals from the disease. People were advised to screen flies out of their homes, to "swat that fly", and to eliminate places for flies to breed.*

Cities directed the chlorination of their water supplies. Hypochlorite of lime was used at first. This was a major step forward in limiting the spread of typhoid. Citizens did not delay this protection by demanding elections as many do now when proposals are made to fluoridate water supplies to prevent dental caries. Subsequently the requirements for sanitary disposal and treatment of sewage aided in control. The practice of chlorination began about 1910. Large outbreaks of typhoid were soon rare. As local health departments were established they investigated cases and contacts, made epidemiolgical studies and instituted control measures. In the twenties and thirties quarantine laws required isolation of the patients and known carriers. A series of negative stool cultures were required before a patient could be released. Health departments enforced these laws. Members of families were also checked to ensure that they were not harboring the bacterial organism (Salmonella typhi) that caused the disease. Those that were free from the organism were released.

The problem lay in tracing the carriers. Most people have heard of "Typhoid Mary", a carrier who infected hundreds of individuals. Regulations prohibited a carrier from engaging in occupations involving the preparation or serving of food, but this was difficult to enforce. Some communities adopted ordinances requiring food personnel to take minimal examinations for specified communicable diseases before issuing cards to permit them to be employed as waiters, waitresses, bakery personnel, dairy workers, or in other food service occupations. The better ordinances required examinations not only for typhoid but also for tuberculosis, and other communicable diseases. Carriers were found through these programs and public health nurses spent considerable time checking cases and documenting carriers. Sometimes these carriers were followed for as many as twenty and twenty-five years. The health department followed one

*What were the symptoms of the disease that caused so much concern? About two weeks after exposure through ingestion of contaminated food, or water, or by hands contaminated with the typhoid organism, patients came down with what seemed like "flu." Severe diarrhea and abdominal pain usually resulted. Children often became ill suddenly and suffered chills and fever. During the second week of the illness a rash on the body, or rose spots, often appeared and the patients became exhausted. This was the most critical period in the course of this serious illness. Intestinal hemorrhages occurred and many persons died in this phase of the disease. Those that survived recovered slowly. We can understand the anxiety and public demand for action. In my own family a two year old brother contracted the disease from raw milk, or contaminated water and died.

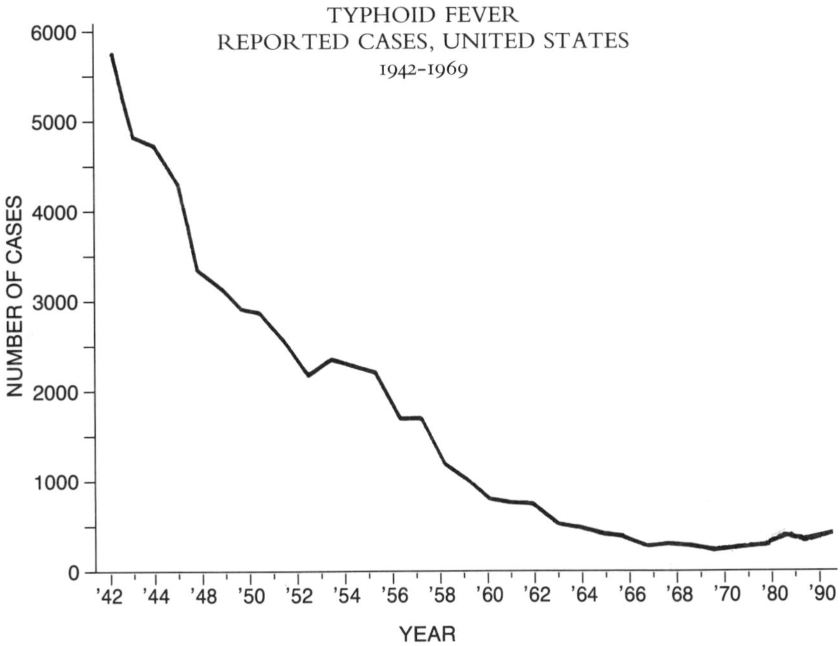
TYPHOID FEVER
REPORTED CASES, UNITED STATES
1942-1969
NUMBER OF CASES
6000
5000
4000
3000
2000
1000
0
'42 '44 '48 '50 '52 '54 '56 '58 '60 '62 '64 '66 '68 '70 '80 '90
YEAR

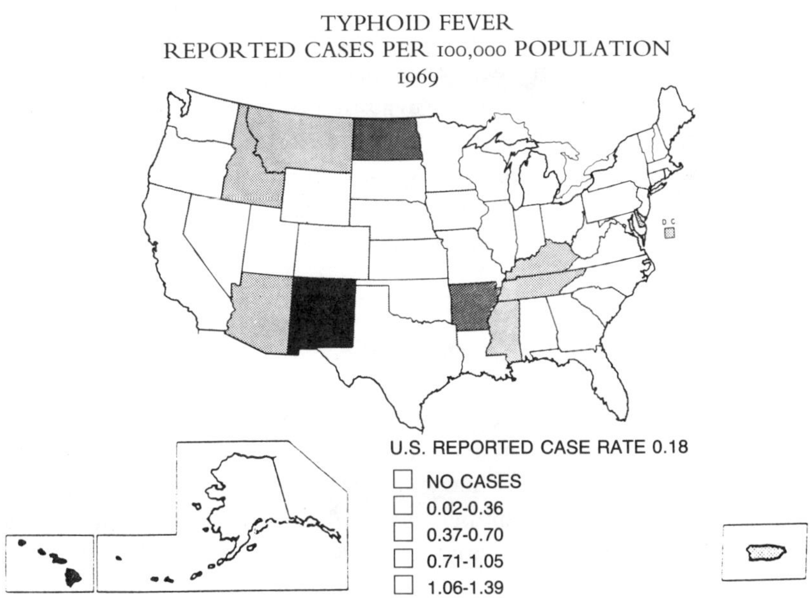
TYPHOID FEVER
REPORTED CASES PER 100,000 POPULATION
1969
D C
U.S. REPORTED CASE RATE 0.18
NO CASES
0.02-0.36
0.37-0.70
0.71-1.05
1.06-1.39

woman in Oregon for fifteen years although she frequently moved from one community to another and was often located in food service occupations. The department persisted; they followed the carrier until finally after gall bladder surgery she had the required numbr of negative cultures showing that she was now free of the infection. She was not permitted to become a "Typhoid Mary". It was in the forties that it was first recognized that typhoid organisms could be harbored in the gall bladder. The treatment at that time of using antibiotics was frequently ineffective in cleaning up the localized infection. In desperation, and to clear themselves of the carrier state, some individuals such as the carrier in Oregon underwent surgical removal of the gall bladder. This was generally successful. Similar control measures were carried out by health departments throughout the country.

The introduction of vaccination against typhoid fever and wide-spread vaccination of those most likely to be exposed, such as men in the military service and individuals traveling in foreign countries was effective.

Some hazards of the disease continue with the existence of unrecognized carriers, the use of untreated surface water for drinking purposes by the uninformed, and the presence of potential cross-connections between potable and contaminated water supplies. An outbreak occured in Zermatt, Switzerland, a small resort city, in the early sixties. It was the result of an accidental "cross-connection". An old sewer line broke contaminating a nearby leaking water line. A temporary drop in pressure in the water main suctioned in contaminated water. Several vacationers from the United States were a part of those infected as a result of drinking the water. Most of them became ill after they had returned to the States. Fortunately all of those exposed were checked out immediately by personnel from the state and local health departments. Treatment and isolation measures were accomplished promptly and the potential outbreak was controlled. Thus the serious hazard of typhoid was largely stamped out.

SMALLPOX

Another of the feared killers was smallpox. It was one of the most infectious diseases ever encountered. In the middle ages in Europe it was known to have destroyed as much as a quarter of the population in a single epidemic. Not only did it kill large numbers of people, but it marked many others horribly, leaving large scars from the pocks that covered the body. There was no treatment for it. People were skeptical of any preventive measure.

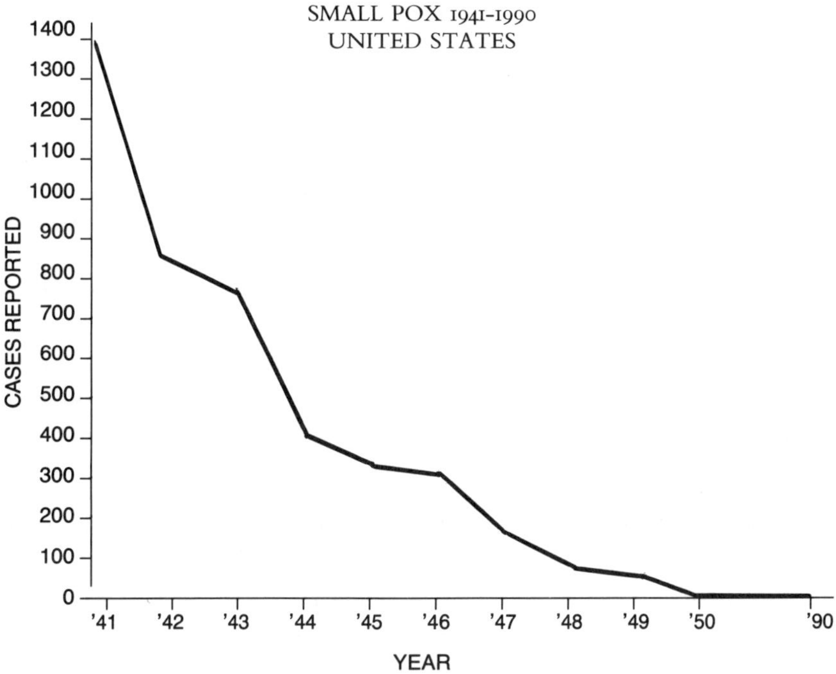

There is little wonder that people panicked when smallpox broke out.

When Edward Jenner, an English physician, in 1796 successfully vaccinated a young boy with cowpox to protect the lad from smallpox, he was initially ridiculed. People expected the boy to grow horns! Physicians and the public were reluctant to accept vaccination. It was necessary for Jenner to publicize his findings in his own pamphlets. Vaccination eventually became accepted, eradication of the disease became possible and the battle began that would finally lead not only to its control but to its complete eradication and disappearance from the world. To accomplish this took time and effort.

Skepticism, fear and superstition about the disease still were prevalent in the latter part of the nineteenth century. Although vaccination against smallpox was done, people usually took advantage of the procedure only when cases were occurring and their fear of contracting the disease was greater than the fear of vaccination. Another motivating factor for vaccination against smallpox was the practice of isolating un-vaccinated persons and denying un-vaccinated children admission to schools.

There was some basis for fearing vaccination. At that time vaccination against smallpox could result not only in very painful swollen arms but in general illness. Vaccines varied in potency. Early vaccination techniques were rugged. An area of the arm, as much as nine square inches, was scarified and a potent vaccine was rubbed on. There was no question of a "take", but the procedure was very rough. Secondary infections were common.

To illustrate, my mother migrated from Norway to the United States about 1900. Vaccination against smallpox was required prior to entry to the United States. To ensure "good protection" the doctor scarified or scraped three wide bars, on her upper arm. The area was then rubbed with the vaccine. About ten days later the wound became markedly inflamed, the entire arm became swollen, and my mother became acutely ill with a severe aching and fever. She was unable to eat. She required bed rest for over a week. Afterwards she had about nine square inches of heavy scarring on her arm. The scar remained with her for the rest of her life. This may have been an unusually severe reaction but one can understand why she and many others feared the procedure. She would not permit her children to be vaccinated against smallpox, even when all school children were required to be vaccinated or stay out of school for two weeks. I was not protected against smallpox until I entered medical school in 1929!

Another hazard to unvaccinated persons was the possibility of contracting the infection in an isolation hospital. They were called "pest houses" by the general public. One of my sisters contracted scarlet fever, was sent to the city of Portland, Oregon, Isolation Hospital for treatment and while there contracted smallpox. This incident occurred in 1920.

As the technique for vaccination and the vaccines were improved through attenuation of the viruses, very little reaction was observed and vaccination generally was accepted. To illustrate, in the late thirties, with intensive educational programs, and strictly on a voluntary basis, 90% of the children in the schools in Wasco County, Oregon, where I served as Director of the Health Department, were protected against the disease. Many of these children had been vaccinated at the age of one year. About 35% to 40% were vaccinated by private physicians and the others in well-baby/well-child conferences. Similar protection was achieved in many areas of the country.

Although it was recommended that immunization preferably be given along with other pediatric care in private physicians' offices, many children did not receive this care. They were vaccinated in health clinics and school vaccination clinics. The multiple pressure technique with lateral pressure of a needle point through a drop of vaccine, usually on the upper arm, was highly effective Children accepted this and many were amused by just enough tickling to produce a freckle.

Occasional outbreaks of smallpox, widely publicizing these cases and fear of the disease, stimulated most parents to take advantage of the readily available vaccinations to protect their children and themselves if they had not recently been vaccinated.

The last cases that I saw in the United States occurred in The Dalles, Oregon. A champion high school football team had just returned from a successful tour. Unfortunately four members of the team were exposed on the trip to someone incubating the smallpox virus. The players picked up the virus as well as their medals. They became seriously ill. As Health Officer, I was called in to confirm the diagnosis and to quarantine the cases.* Rigid quarantine was maintained, thousands of possible contacts were vaccinated and happily there were no secondary cases.

In a neighboring small county, although the cases were never officialy reported, it was said that about fifty cases of smallpox had occurred in the same year. In 1938, another incident related to smallpox occurred while I was Health Officer in The Dalles. Dr. James Odell, Director of the Eastern Oregon State Tuberculosis Hospital, called me to see one of the recently admitted patients who had developed a small pock on his face. He had been vaccinated against smallpox. However, I vividly remembered the report of a serious outbreak in England where a military man returning from a foreign assignment had a small lesion on his face. It was thought to be an acne pustule as he too had been vaccinated against smallpox. In actuality it was a smallpox lesion. The officer served as a carrier. About ten days after his return members of his family and several contacts became ill with smallpox. This was a very virulent form of the disease. Before the outbreak in England was controlled several deaths had occurred. This recollection may have biased our judgement. We were aware of the fact that the man had possibly been exposed to chickenpox. There had also

*Each of the young men complained most about severe headaches and pain in their backs. They said it felt as if their backs were broken. This was characteristic of early smallpox. They did have fever and general malaise and the initial pimple-like, papular rash developed into a host of small, umbilicated pustular, "aspirin tablet" size lesions. Three of the athletes had them mostly on the trunk of the body with only a few lesions on the face. One of the players was very ill and was covered with pocks. Luckily, all recovered with minimal scarring.

been a few cases of smallpox in the state at that time. Not wishing to be responsible for an outbreak similar to that which occurred in England, and out of concern for the patients, I recommended vaccination for all non-vaccinated patients. Dr. Odell said, "Fine! How about you doing it?" I agreed that I would. One of my staff nurses and I spent most of the day vaccinating patients. Fortunately there were no cases and no complications. After these many years I still am not certain what the diagnosis was, but I think that under the circumstances I would still have done the vaccinations.

We did recognize two forms of smallpox. The outbreak in The Dalles was mild and of a type which we called "Cuban Itch." Very few people died from this form of the disease.

A much more malignant type (Hemorrhagic Smallpox) resulting in hemorrhages of the skin and bleeding throughout the body, often resulted in death. An epidemic of this kind broke out in Minnesota in the winter of 1924-25. There were approximately 1,000 cases and 300 deaths in Minneapolis alone. Fortunately this type of the disease was rare in the United States, only occaisionaly being "carried" in from Asia, or Africa. In the early thirties, several people died in a small outbreak in Chicago. I recall only two other instances of this kind, one in the forties to which I referred earlier, occurring in England, and a similar episode in the fifties at Fort Lewis, Washington. A returning soldier, previously vaccinated suffered a mild, unusual form of the disease. It was due to a malignant form of the virus and some fifteen or sixteen people became ill. Again, some died before the outbreak could be brought under control.

My wife and I spent two years in India from 1966 to 1968, during which time I saw many cases of smallpox in the villages and heard of many more. In one village with a population of about one thousand it was estimated that over four hundred cases of smallpox had occurred in one year. The village "vaccinator" had for several years neglected his job of vaccinating the infants and when the virus was brought in, it spread rapidly thorugh the village. Most of these cases were not officially reported. As an aside, we heard that the "vaccinator" had collected his paycheck monthly.

In the United States only one case of smallpox has occurred in recent years. That was the result of a laboratory accident when a virulent smallpox virus was taken out of storage in a laboratory freezer. Freezing had not affected its potency.

The total elimination of smallpox is a marvelous accomplishment in the annals of Public Health. Local Health Departments had a major role in control in the United States.

BUBONIC PLAGUE*

Another scourge was bubonic plague. It is a pestilence which was greatly feared because those who contracted it were almost certain to die. Its explosive spread through Europe in the nineteenth century is well-documented. Because the infection was transmitted to humans by fleas from infected rats, the disease was most likely to break out around port cities where rats from foreign ports deserted the ships.

The first case to be recognized in the United States was found in San Francisco, California, in March 1900. One of the residents of the Chinese section was found dead from the disease. The City Board of Health that had confirmed the diagnosis placed the entire Chinese population under quarantine with the area roped off and police on guard. Imagine the uproar! It became an intense political issue. The Board of Health, local and state health officials and the USMHS were severely attacked verbally, as was the Mayor. Appeals were made to the Governor of California. Lawsuits were filed in an attempt to prevent the Marine Hospital Service from enforcing quarantine at the port. Political pressures were applied. Health officials and the mayor stood firm in the face of the deluge of public criticism and attacks, much of which would be considered libelous today. A special commission of outstanding experts was appointed by the USMHS Surgeon General despite the protests of the Governor. The Commision members observed six cases of unquestionable plague within a few days of their arrival. On announcing their findings the opposition melted. The Governor asked the federal government to take charge of the Plague Control Program. It is interesting to note that the Association of State and Territorial Health Officers informed representatives of California that other

---

*This is a serious disease caused by an infection with a bacteria Pasteurella pestis. The latter infects rodents—rats and squirrels—and is transmitted by fleas from rodent to rodent, hence to man. Infection in rats is most hazardous to man as rats invade spaces used by man. If a human is bitten and inoculated by an infected flea, the bacteria invade the lymphatics and are carried through them to the lymph nodes. The latter become inflamed and enlarge to form what at called "buboes" from which the disease gets its name. With this invasion an individual suddenly becomes critically ill with total exhaustion, high fever, and a generalized aching and pain. If the bacteria invade the blood stream and spread throughout the body, pneumonia or meningitis may occur. Either generally are fatal unless antibiotics are given early. Patients with bubonic plague pneumonia can transmit the disease to others by droplets from the lungs.

states would take drastic action against California unless adequate control measures were instituted. Control was continued until 1905 when it was thought that the threat was over. It was not! One year after the great San Francisco earthquake and fire of 1906, it broke out again. There were one hundred and sixty cases and seventy-seven deaths before the plague was checked. This time the politicians and the press cooperated. They had learned to respect the health departments during the first outbreak.

Sporadic cases have occurred in coastal cities since. Fear of Bubonic Plague is such that cities are willing to expend millions of dollars to rat proof buildings and to otherwise control the rodents when Plague-infected rats are found. This was seen in Oakland and Los Angeles, California in 1924.

The most serious threat more recently was in Tacoma, Washington. One hundred and nine plague infected rats were found in the city between 1942 and 1944. There were no human cases. The port was closed to shipping for many months until the rat population could be brought under control. In eastern Oregon, Washington, California, and other states where ground squirrels abound, evidence that these rodents harbor fleas infected with the pasteurella pestis that causes plague, can be found at any time if one looks for them. Isolated cases of infection in man can, and do occur, but the hazard of infection from ground squirrels is relatively slight as they ordinarily do not invade homes as rats do. Early recognition of the disease in rodents (and man), and prompt measures to limit spread are essential to control bubonic plague.

LEPROSY

Another pestilence that was much dreaded, has been known for centuries. It has occurred in much of the world, but its mode of spread is not yet fully understood. That disease is leprosy, or Hansen's disease. Caused by a bacterium, Hansen's bacillus, it has a long incubation period of four or five years, and, unless treated, is fatal in fifteen, or twenty years. It most commonly starts in childhood. Most of the cases in the United States occurred in the South. Hawaii likewise was troubled by the disease. There were not many cases in the continental United States but there was a sufficient number to warrant establishing a national Leprosarium at Carville, Louisiana, where lepers could to sent to live and receive treatment. There is a second one in Hawaii. After successful medical treatment, limiting progress of the disease, patients were often discharged to receive continued treatment and supervision in their own communities. Registration, and strict follow-up was, and still is, maintained. A few cases yet occur. Fear of this disease which prevailed in the middle ages, is reflected in the structure of some of the older buildings. In visiting an old Stav Kirche (Stave Church) in the mountains of Norway, we were intrigued by the strangeness of the structure. It looked somewhat like a Chinese Pagoda with an inner and an outer wall three to four feet apart. This created a walkway around the high ceilinged, one room church. The roof was made of long stavs or shakes, blackened by age. Near the back of the church there was an opening in the inner wall. When the guide was asked what the opening was for, he explained that when the church was built, about 1000, or 1100 A.D., there were a number of lepers in the area. Because of fear of the disease, lepers were not permitted in the sanctuary. They were allowed to walk through the passageway surrounding the sanctuary, past the opening in the inner wall. At this point the priest could see and bless them through the opening.

Today the dread, suspicion, and fear have largely been dispelled as a result of successful treatment and education. The Lepromin skin test, similar to a test for tuberculosis, is now used to detect the tuberculoid type, a milder form of the disease. Techniques in culturing the organism have made early and accurate diagnosis a reality. A major breakthrough in treatment occurred in Carville, in 1941, when Dr. Guy H. Fuget, a Public Health Service Officer, introduced the sulphones in treatment. Dopsone used together with Rifampin was quite effective. Although the usefulness of these drugs was not immediatly apparent in the patients, the final results were spectacular in stabalizing and preventing extension of the disease. New antibiotics are even more effective than sulphones.

It is worthy to note that much of the disfigurement in loss of fingers, toes, and scarring of the body was due to injury rather than the disease process. Suffering from nerve involvement and loss of sensation, a person with the disease could experience a severe burn, an injury, or a series of injuries resulting in disfigurement, with-out any awareness or pain at the time of the injury.

Leprosy which caused so much crippling, disfigurement, isolation, and even the banishment of those suffering from it, has been largely controlled in the developed world through advances in medical science, treatment, and through public health measures.

EPIDEMIC MENINGITIS*

In the early part of this century another greatly feared and generally fatal disease was called "spinal meningitis." We now recognize several kinds of meningitis including meningoccus, tuberculous, syphilitic, strepococcal, staphylococcal, pneumococcal, and those due to an influenza virus, other viruses and fungus infections. The most common and the most feared in earlier years was that due to the meningococcus. It is the latter that causes epidemic meningitis. The disease was feared because it was so often fatal within days. There was no specific treatment. Infants, children, and young people were more frequently attacked than adults and many died of it before the introduction of sulpha drugs and antibiotics. It was known that about twenty percent or more of our population, although apparently well, were carriers harboring the organsims in their nasal passages. The spread of the disease was predominantly due to these carriers, rather than to actual cases.

Many sero-groups and even more sero-types have been found in recent years. They vary in virulence, tendency to invade the blood streams, and in their resistance to drugs and antibiotics. It is interesting that organisms of one group may change virulence, resistance to antibiotics, invasive ability, and other characteristics. There is much variation in the resistance of individuals to the organisms.

Before sulphonamides and antibiotics, very little could be done for these patients. I remember seeing and caring for some of them at Doernbecher Children's Hospital in Portland, Oregon, in the early thirties. One felt very helpless to see these seriously ill babies and little children, heads drawn back, spastic, and often unconscious, and realize that all you could do for them was to give supportive treatment. The diagnosis was confirmed by doing a spinal tap and analyzing the spinal fluid. Body fluids were maintained with intravenous, or subcutaneous solutions. All cases were strictly isolated.

Diagnosis was important because patients with meningitis complicating mumps, measles, or other childhood infections were much more likely to recover.

The introduction of Sulphonamides in the mid-thirties dramatically

---

*The first indications of infection are severe headache, chills and fever, nausea and vomiting, stiffness of the neck and back and general prostration. A minute hemorrhagic type of rash often appeared on the body. Mental confusion, delirium, convulsions, and lapses into unconsciousness usually precede death in untreated cases.

changed the outlook for these patients. With prompt diagnosis, early treatment with adequate doses of sulphonamide, and continued supportive treatment, these patients now speedily improved and usually recovered. They became fully conscious, able to eat and drink, and were soon up and around. It was said that in developing countries a missionary with a sack of sulpha drugs could miraculously cure individuals with meningitis merely by passing out the pills.

Major recorded epidemics of the disease occurred in 1929, 1936, and in 1943. Occasional sporadic cases have occurred since. There has been an apparent slight increase in recent years. In the past when a case was found in a school child, health departments checked on the contacts in school and at home. Any child suspected of coming down with the disease was isolated, nose and throat cultures were taken, and prophylactic treatment with sulphonamides was given.

The most threatening outbreaks that have occurred in more recent years generally have been found in Induction Centers of the military. In 1965 while I was serving as Acting-Director of Health for the State of California, our department became concerned about a number of cases of epidemic meningitis that were occurring at Fort Ord, California. Thousands of young recruits were being brought in for basic training. Our department was called for assistance to control the outbreak. We sent an epidemiologist to Fort Ord. In cooperation with the Fort's medical staff, every aspect of the outbreak was scrutinized and carefully studied. Additional precautions were recommended. Nose and throat cultures of all new recruits were taken. Prophylactic treatment was instituted. Rigorous excercise was curtailed. The number of recruits per barrack was reduced and beds were re-arranged to minimize airborn transmission between recruits.

When these measures failed, (and because civilians were also becoming infected with the disease), visitation by friends and relatives was curtailed. Sadly, deaths occurred within the military and in the nearby civilian population. Within the military, only the new recruits were involved. After several months of futile efforts to control the outbreak, and with press, radio, television, and the public clamoring for action, our department concluded that the only means of stopping the outbreak was to halt the flow of recruits to Fort Ord for at least three months. We realized that this was a radical recommendation with serious implications for the Army, but we concluded that we should urge the action.

The need for training military personnel and the importance of Fort

Ord in that training was very great. Only the most serious of problems could necessitate interruption even for three months. Surgeon General of the Army, Leonard D. Heaton, flew to San Francisco to discuss the proposal. He and I boarded an Army "Jet Star" plane. We flew to Los Angeles where we conferred with the then Governor Pat Brown. We agreed that such a drastic step must be taken. General Heaton and I then flew to Fort Ord whre we met with the commanding officers and medical staff of the Fort to inform them of the decision. Reluctantly, this action was taken. No further recruits were trained at Fort Ord for many months and no further cases of meningitis occurred at the Fort or in the surrounding civilian population.

For several years sulphonamide therapy was effective, but the success of that "magic treatment" began to fade. Today, antibiotics are used almost exclusively to treat epidemic meningitis as the meningococcic bacteria have become Sulpha resistant. A vaccine for some sero-groups is now available and is being used to protect new recruits from meningococcus meningitis. Research on this disease continues. This previously fatal affliction is yielding to health science and control measures.

DIPHTHERIA*

Diphtheria was a merciless killer in the early part of this century. It was greatly feared, and rightly so, as it could devastate families. In my mother's family four of five of her brothers and sisters succumbed to the disease in early childhood. At that time there was no known treatment or immunization for the disease. It was very infectious.

Diphtheria had been known for centuries. In fact, it was clearly described by Arteur in the first century A.D. Spread by carriers who did not suffer from the symptoms, and by persons who were ill with the disease, it attacked hundreds of thousands of persons over the centuries and at times crushed whole families. It was particularly severe in the late 1600's killing thousands of people. Imagine the panic engendered in families. One could

*Ordinarily diphtheria is characterized by sore throat, fever, and generalized flu-like symptoms with characteristic yellow, or grey patches on the tonsils and mucous membranes of the nose and throat. Clinically, one of the criteria of diagnosis was bleeding if an attempt was made to remove the false leathery membrane. Toxin produced by the bacteria in the nose and throat spread throughout the body often affecting the nervous system, heart, kidneys, and intestinal tract. Unless antitoxin was given promptly and in sufficient quantity, death could occur within six to ten days due to obstruction of the trachea and pharynx, the toxemia, or heart failure.

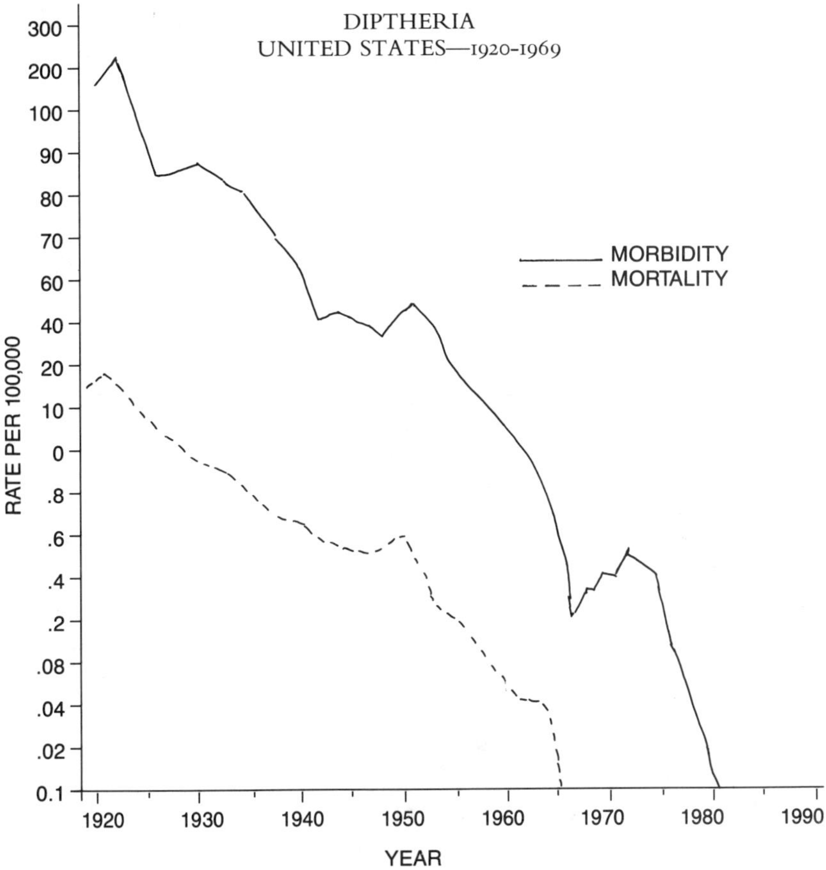

avoid persons who were ill, but what could one do about individuals who appeared well but who harbored those deadly germs and could infect others resulting in serious illness or death? What caused it? A curse? An "ill wind?'

Refinement of the microscope and improved culture techniques made it possible to determine the causative agent, which previously had not been known. In 1899 Klebs and Loeffler described what we now know as the Klebs-Loeffler bacillus as the cause of the disease. Soon after this antitoxin was developed by injecting the toxin of diphtheria into horses who developed antitoxin, collecting their serum, and treating patients with diphtheria by injecting the antitoxin. This saved many lives. Real prevention began when Bela Schick, an Austrian physician, developed a skin test in 1913 to determine the presence or absence of immunity to diphtheria.

Persons shown not to be immune could then be given toxin—antitoxin, or toxoid, to stimulate the development of immunity. Public acceptance of immunizations did not occur until the late twenties and early thirties.

In these years millions of children were Schick tested and immunized against diphtheria. With the establishment of more local health departments in the late thirties, staffs of these departments, cooperating with schools and private physicians on a voluntary basis, protected 65-70% of the school children. Babies and pre-school children were being protected by private physicians and by health departments in well-baby and pre-school clinics.

In the early forties some states adopted laws requiring all children entering school for the first time to be protected against diphtheria and smallpox. Development of toxoid, a modified diphtheria toxin, made it possible to immunize adults and a greater number of older children with relatively little reaction.

With these protective measures and strict quarantine of diagnosed cases and identified diphtheria carriers, incidence in United States rapidly decreased but occasional outbreaks did occur usually in areas where immunization had been neglected. A good illustration of this was the occurrence in the early forties of diphtheria in a small Oregon community. Thirty cases were reported before the outbreak was controlled. It was an "explosive" type of occurence with a number of persons falling ill within a period of a few days. An investigation revealed that the community had only three small dairies. All sold only raw, unpasteurized milk. Although each had about an equal number of customers, the majority of the families with diphtheria obtained their milk from one of the dairies. A study of this dairy revealed that the dairyman's wife who helped bottle and cap the milk, had been ill and had a very sore throat about ten days earlier. She had recovered, but a young high school student who also helped in bottling and capping the raw milk had a slight sore throat. Throat cultures from the farmer and his wife were negative but the high school student had positive nose and throat cultures for diphtheria. The dairy was immediatly closed and the family was quarantined until repeated cultures taken from the student were negative. All residents of the community had been advised to pasteurize their milk at home in addition to being immunized. Unfortunately, the wife of one of the city officials contracted the disease and died of it.

The health department recommended that all milk sold by dairies be pasteurized to avoid such infections including scarlet fever, septic soar throat, undulant fever, typhoid fever, tuberculosis, and salmonellosis.

Opponents of pasteurization charged that we had "manufactured" the diphtheria outbreak to support a pasteurization program. They took their complaints to the legislature. The hard facts soon quelled their attack.

Another outbreak occurring in the fifties was very serious, not as much because the of the number of cases, but as a result of the virulence of the diphtheria organism. The cases broke out in southern Oregon, chiefly in Josephine and Jackson counties. The outbreak was termed "Bull neck" diphtheria because of the severity of the infection and the marked swelling of the throat.

In this outbreak cases prevailed in persons who gave histories of previous immunizations to diphtheria. It is possible that they may have never received the required number of "shots" to complete the immunization. Those attacked became critically ill, had massive swelling in the neck, and some of the children did not respond to treatment and died. Unusually large doses of antitoxin were required to combat this particularly virulent infection.

There were some benefits. As so often happens, because of the great fear engendered by such an outbreak, large numbers of children and adults who had neglected their immunizations or who were only partially protected, crowded in to private physicians offices and health department clinics for immunization.

Throughout the United States the incidence of diphtheria has continued to decline. However, seven hundred and fifty-one cases of diphtheria were reported to the Communicable Disease Center in Atlanta, Georgia, during the period 1971 through 1975. Thirty-six percent of these cases were in persons twenty years of age or older. Forty-two respiratory cases occurred in the Seattle, Washington, area during this period and over two hundred cases of what was previously thought to be a rare type of the disease, dermatological diphtheria, were reported in Alaska. This caused a real concern as many "old timers" remembered when Nome, Alaska, had been ravaged by diphtheria in 1925. That outbreak was widespread. People recollected the use of dog teams to rush antitoxin to isolated areas.

More recently there has been an outbreak of diphthteria on the eastern seaboard. It is hoped that through more complete protection of the entire population with immunizations against diphtheria the disease can be, like smallpox, completely eradicated. The existence of individuals in the carrier state of the disease makes this more difficult.

YELLOW FEVER*

Epidemics of this disease were largely limited to the southern states. It was one of the major pestilences imported from other countries that terrorized people when it emerged. In 1878, an epidemic swept through Louisiana, Mississippi, Tennnessee, Alabama, and other southern states. The crew of a tugboat headed from New Orleans to Pittsburgh, helped spread contagion. Twenty-three of the crew died. The infection was carried to many communities. Grenada, Mississippi, was devastated by this epidemic. Most of the 2,200 inhabitants fled. Imagine the magnitude of the panic that would cause people to give up their homes. Fear of a tornado or hurricane could not have been greater. Of the estimated two hundred stalwarts who remained, practically all died.

An outbreak occurred in Franklin, Louisiana, in 1898. There were six hundred seven cases and nine deaths. It ended in late October just before the first killing frost. The last outbreak of yellow fever in the United States erupted in New Orleans in 1905. It lasted from July until late October. The Public Health and Marine Hospital Service was asked to assume control. Almost 3,500 people became ill of whom approximately four-hundred and fifty died. Mosquito control proved to be effective in this outbreak.

In 1881, Dr. Carlos Finlay, was the first to suggest that the Aedes aegypti mosquito might be responsible for carrying the disease. It was Dr. Henry R. Carter of the USMHS in 1898 who demonstrated that the mosquito was not infectious for about twelve days after feeding on a person with the disease. This was a significant finding. It was later discovered that the monkey could serve as an intermediary host. It remained for Dr. Walter Reed, heading an Army Board, and based on results of experiments using volunteers in Cuba in 1900 and 1901, to prove beyond a doubt that yellow fever was transmitted by the Aedes aegypti mosquito, and that the disease was due to a virus. Ironically, Dr. Reed died on November 23, 1902, in Washington, D.C., not from yellow fever, but from peritonitis after an appendectomy.

The major problem after the disease was brought under control in the United States was to prevent its re-introduction. After the Spanish American War, some 30,000 troops returning from Cuba were inspected for yellow

---

*This viral disease characterized by a recurrent fever, prostration, general body pain, hemorrhages of nose, mouth, and skin, jaundice, and finally delirium in the more severe forms is often fatal.

fever and many were quarantined for five days to assure that none were ill with the disease.

In 1937 the United States Public Health Service assigned Dr. Mason V. Hargett to Miami, Florida to activate a yellow fever control program. This was due to the fact that a number of cases of the disease had been found there, outbreaks that probably resulted because Miami was the point of entry for the majority of airplanes from South America, and because the Aedes aegypti mosquito was prevalent in the swamps around the city. Persons leaving the United States for areas with the disease and airline personnel were offered vaccination. Planes were sprayed with pyrethrum, an insecticide, and after passengers and crew disembarked, a minute search of arriving planes was made for insects. A mosquito control program was initiated in the Miami area. A cadre of public health personnel was vaccinated against yellow fever. This staff was available for control if the need arose. Fortunately this threat did not materialize.

In the meantime, various types of vaccine were developed. In 1941, the production of a vaccine was begun at the Rocky Mountain Laboratory in Hamilton, Montana. A live attenuated virus, serum free, vaccine was found to be safe and 100% effective. This type was the only kind produced after 1942. The only cases reported in the United States since that date have been in a few individuals who contracted the disease in another country. In effect, one of the most feared diseases at the turn of the century was brought under control in the United States as a result of good epidemiology and in promptly instituting effective public health control measures. Only travelers in the tropics now need to be concerned with yellow fever.

THE CONQUEST OF MALARIA*

The conquest of malaria, commonly called ague, or Marsh Fever, is further proof of the effectiveness of public health measures. The disease had been recognized in the tropics for centuries. Cinchona bark had been used

*The disease was somewhat unusual in that an individual suffered periodic attacks of headache, chills, fever, nausea, and vomiting. Episodes lasted six to eight hours during the time of exodus of parasites from the blood cells which they had invaded. This occurred every three days (tertian), or four days (quartan), depending on the type of parasite. Between episodes, the individual could feel well. Jaundice often developed. In the most severe cases, due to P. falciparum, complications, including dark discoloration of the urine (termed black water fever), could result in early death.

for treatment for over two hundred years although quinine, an extract of the bark, was not produced as a drug until the early nineteenth century.

It was known that there were at least four types of plasmodia, the infectious agent, the most common in the United States, being P. vivax and P. falciparum. A fifth, occuring in the other parts of the world was recognized later. Although the disease primarily occurs in man, it was found in some areas of the world, to be transmissable by mosquitos from monkeys to man and from man to monkeys, as well as from man to man.

Malaria was appearing in the United States particularly in the warmer, moister, southern states. It was estimated that around the turn of the century about two to three thousand deaths occurred each year in this country. Little attention was given to it until about 1912. The USPHS became concerned and in 1914 asked Congress for funds to survey the disease. About $16,000.00 was made available.

In making the survey it was found that along one of the lengthy railroads in the south, physicians reported that half of their practice consisted of treating patients with malaria. Although not in epidemic form, it was determined that occurrence of the disease extended to isolated areas in states as far north as Oregon and Michigan. I remember a few cases occurring each summer in the hop fields near Salem, Oregon. Migrants from southern states came to pick hops. Some probably were malaria carriers, and we did have Anopheles (mosquitos) in the area.

Ronald Ross in 1897-1899, working in India, discovered that the Anopheles carried the Plasmodia from a person infected with the malarial parasite to another person. This could only occur after several days of incubation of the protozoa in the mosquito. An infected person could not directly infect another person. This discovery was a vital one in efforts to control the disease.

The USPHS teams found that screening of houses and giving quinine to householders would reduce the number of carriers by as much as two-thirds. Later, stimulated by the necessity of controlling malaria around military training camps in the south during World War I (1914-1919), swamps were drained, oil and a larvacide, Paris green, were used to prevent Anopheline mosquito from breeding in areas extending one mile from the camps (the distance the mosquito was known to travel). These measures were highly successful. After the first World War, similar control measures were adoptd in many communities of the south through the joint efforts of the USPHS and state and local health departments. When DDT became available it was used in dusting homes. Chlordane, in later years was also found to be useful in controlling mosquitoes. These measures and education of the residents of the area to the hazards and means of control were very effective. By 1950, relatively few cases occurred and most of these were imported.

Beginning in 1942 the USPHS conducted studies on drugs other than quinine for treatment and suppression of malaria. Over 2500 compounds were tested. After tests on over four hundred volunteers it was concluded that Chloraquine was the most useful drug. Not only was it effective in treatment, but it was found that 0.5 grams given weekly and for twelve weeks after an individual left an endemic area (one in which malaria was occurring), would prevent infection in an exposed person. This discovery was invaluable in World War II. Japan had shut off the supply of quinine from Java, the chief source of cinchona bark. Although stock-piling and conservation for the military had been carried out, a shortage developed. The availability of Chloraquine was life-saving.

With this knowledge and control measures instituted by health departments the disease has largely been eliminated from the United States.

TYPHUS FEVER*

This is another of the great pestilences that killed millions of people in foreign countries and that accounted for thousands of deaths among U.S. troops in World War I. Happily it did not gain a foothold in the United States. Small outbreaks occurred in Philiadelphia in 1883 and in New York in 1891 and 1892. A minor epidemic of typhus fever broke out in New Mexico in 1921. Sporadic mild cases occurred in Alabama and Georgia in the early twenties.

Dr. Kenneth F. Maxcy did the basic epidemiology on typhus fever. I was fortunate in being one of his students at Johns Hopkins School of Public Health. Drs. Herald R. Cox, Norman H. Topping, and Ida A. Bengston of the Rocky Mountain Laboratory and National Institute of Health

*The disease was often mistaken for typhoid fever as its symptoms were similar except for a more abrupt onset, termination and, the skin rash. It was confused with Rocky Mountain Spotted Fever. Typhus fever is a disease caused by one of the Rickettsiae, a minute, usually intra-cellular micro-organism, larger than a virus. The more severe type of the disease, louse-born (by the so-called "cootie') was prevalent during World War I and at times of famine, prior to discovery of the cause. A milder form transmitted to humans by the flea of the rat, was not very serious.

developed an effective vaccine that protected thousands of our troops during World War II. Vaccination, control of body lice, rats and fleas, and measures developed in the first half of this century conquered this plague which had ravaged peoples of other lands for hundreds of years.

POLIOMYELITS (INFANTILE PARALYSIS)

Polio, infantile paralyisis, or "anterior poliomyelitis" was first recognized and eventually controlled in the United States, during this century.

Polio has been of particular interest to me because I have seen so many children and adults suddenly stricken by the virus, almost completely paralyzed, some encased in huge white plaster casts, many doomed to lie enclosed in confining respirators for weeks, while others died despite heroic efforts to save them. Over the years I have observed improvements in treatment, substitution of physical therapy for the casts, development of the vaccines, the launching of trial programs to test them, the massive programs to protect our entire population against the disease, and the near elimination of it. This has been one of the most inspiring experiences of my life.

It seems strange that polio was not previously recognized. There is some evidence of occurrence of the disease in ancient Egypt. Did it disappear for a time? Was it over-shadowed by the "plagues"? Was it a new disease? If so, where did it come from? Now some believe that it was occurring in infants and was called "Summer Sickness". Immunity developed in infancy usually protected adults. Adults living on a Swedish Isle apparently lacked this immunity, and the first outbreak of polio in adults was recognized there. Little was known about polio, its cause, mode of spread, or how to treat it when it was first recognized. It was known to be communicable, but how? Although it was called infantile paralysis, it was rather rare in tiny infants. They apparently received immunity from their mothers. It did attack children most commonly, probably after loss of their immunity. Adults were sometimes afflicted. As the name implies, paralysis of extremities was most characteristic of the disease. In extreme cases, respiratory paralysis occurred. Because virtually nothing was known about the control of the disease, and treatment in earlier years was ineffective, people were fearful of polio. This fear was apparent in appeals for public financial support of Polio research and care. Placards, showing the picture of a crippled child, proclaimed, "Is Your Child Next?" The fatality rate was high—

PARALYTIC POLIOMYELITIS
GEOGRAPHIC DISTRIBUTION, UNITED STATES, 1972

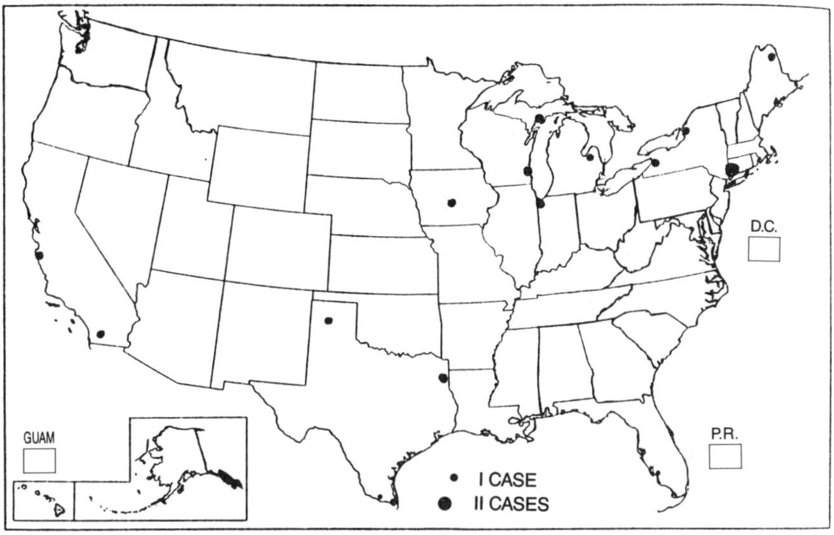

PARALYTIC POLIOMYELITIS—
REPORTED CASES BY MONTH, UNITED STATES, 1962-1972

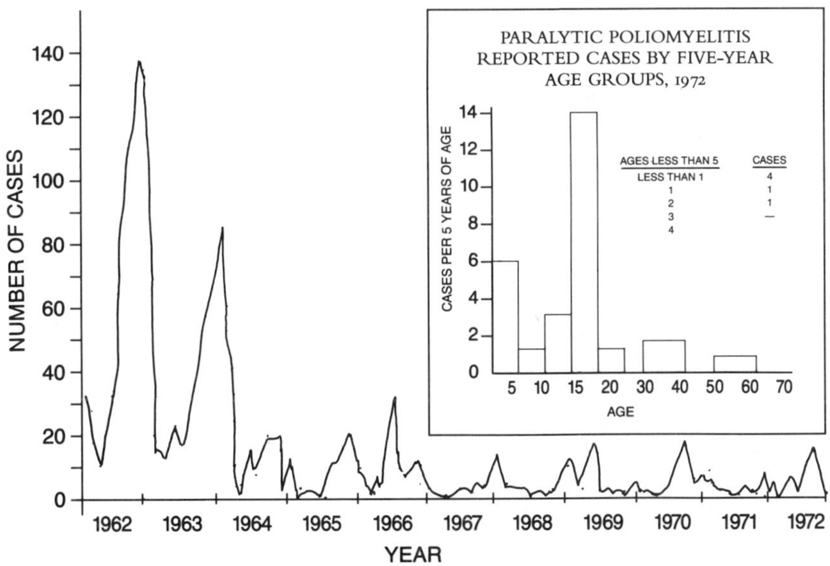

POLIOMYLITIS (PARALYTIC) — BY YEAR, UNITED STATES, 1951-1989

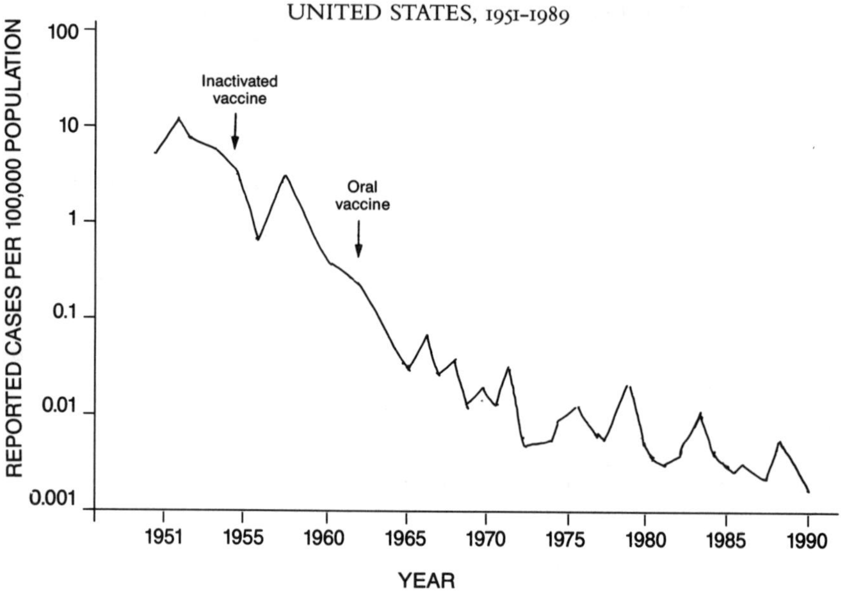

about one in every five afflicted. Prior to 1930, when respirators were first used, the unfortunate who developed respiratory paralysis usually succumbed rapidly.

The first known epidemic of infantile paralysis in the United States occurred in the summer of 1907. As mentioned an outbreak on an isolated island off the coast of Sweden had been reported earlier. Our first cases appeared in states along the Atlantic coast. The disease re-appeared in a localized epidemic in the New York City area in 1909. By this time cases were being recognized in many parts of the United States as well as in Europe. It was in this year that Drs. Simon Flexner and Paul A. Lewis, at the Rockefeller Institute for Medical Research, demonstrated a virus from afflicted humans as the cause and successfully transmitted the virus from afflicted humans to monkeys. Monkeys had been inoculated with polio in Germany earlier in that year.

My first recollection of seeing a case of polio was at Doernbecher Children's Memorial Hospital in Portland, Oregon, in 1932. I was a junior in medical school. Dr. J. B. Bilderback, the "grandfather of pediatrics" in the Pacific Northwest, had a patient, a nine year old boy with bulbar polio, (paralysis of the respiratory center). Dr. Bilderback presented the case to our class. The boy was in an adult size respirator. He was the first patient at Doernbecher to be treated in a respirator. Although we were only students, we realized that without the aide of the machine to literally breathe for the young patient, he would die. This young boy survived.*

In visiting the polio wards it was impressive and somewhat depressing to see paralyzed youngsters in heavy plaster casts, many of them encasing the childs entire body, with the exception of the head. Arms and legs extended in a huge X-type formation similar to the distress postion assumed in signalling for help in an emergency. Ropes and pulleys attached to frames over the beds were used to suspend limbs and to assist in turning patients.

To me, the encouraging part of the experience was to see many of these youngsters, encased as they were, smile and chat with each other, and later recover. What patience. Seldom was a cry ever heard and then only from a small child when parents, all in masks and white isolation gowns, were leaving on Sunday afternoon, the only day during the entire week when visitors were permitted.

---

*This episode was indelibly stamped on my memory when a few years later I learned that the young nurse who took care of this historical case was to become my wife.

It is interesting to speculate how this treatment in casts developed as the benefit of active treatment had been recognized early. In 1906 an article appeared in the Journal of the American Medical Association outlining treatment for infantile paralysis. It stated:

> The following general means are employed:
> 1. Massage and warm clothing.
> 2. Electricity: both galvanism and faradism.*
> 3. Functional use as far as possible.
> 4. Passive motion of each joint to its full range daily.
> 5. A light night brace if the extremity lies in anabnormal position during sleep.
>
> *(alternating or direct current)

Apparently, this course of treatment had not generally been adopted or it had been forgotten or modified. Casting became the accepted treatment.

About 1935 Sister Kenny, an Australian nurse, toured the United States broadcasting her success in treating polio patients with hot packs and massage. She gave live demonstrations of her methods. The packs were massive. They consisted of heavy woolen blankets dipped in tubs of very hot water and wrung out using old-fashioned clothes wringers (two compression rubber rollers operated by a hand crank or motor). Massage was vigorous. Foot and hand supports were used. Physicians, particularly orthopedic surgeons, were initially skeptical of Sister Kenny's treatment fearing crippling contractures. Many openly opposed it. Gradually however, the superiority of the revived treatment over cast treatment techniques was proven and children and adults were freed from casts.

Following this change, and the utilization of respirators when needed, very little further advance in treatment occurred, except for surgical correction of persistent orthopedic deformities. As the mode of spread of the virus was unknown, effective preventive measures could not be taken. In epidemics, schools were sometimes closed chiefly because of the concern of parents. As public swimming pools were thought to be a possible means of spreading the infections, they too, were often closed during epidemics. Chlorination of water supplies was carefully supervised. In 1952 about four hundred cases of polio were reported in Oregon. California, with ten times the population of Oregon, recorded almost 4,000 cases the same year. Not all cases were reported as many were very mild and were not seen by physicians. It was observed that the large majority of cases occurred during the summer and early fall months. This supported the idea that the disease was more like typhoid, first involving the intestinal tract. Respiratory infections were more prone to occur in winter months. The means by which an infecting agent reached the nervous system was not known.

Polio could strike suddenly and progress very rapidly. I remember one of our neighbors, a young mother about thirty years of age. She had planned a weekend trip with her husband, but on Friday afternoon, she developed a rather severe headache and tenseness of the neck. She called a physician, another neighbor, who examined her. He could not make a definitive diagnosis, but recommended that she postpone her trip. He suggested rest and fluids. The next day she was worse with pain in her back. A chiropractic physician was called in. He "adjusted" her spine. Unfortunatly her symptoms became more severe and she had difficulty in moving. That evening the physician-surgeon hospitalized her. She was diagnosed as having polio, isolated, and was carefully observed. On Sunday morning she developed respiratory paralysis and was placed in a respirator. Sunday evening she sank into a deep coma and died, leaving behind a woe-stricken husband and three children.

One can easily understand the fear resulting from such cases. Residual paralysis and crippling were also feared. One of the well-known victims of polio was Franklin Delano Roosevelt. He contracted the disease in adulthood and suffered severe paralysis and atrophy of his legs. He was forced to use a wheelchair for a great part of his adult life. Because of his interest in polio, Roosevelt, who became the thirty-second President of the United States, actively promoted the March of Dimes to support the work of the National Foundation for Infantile Paralysis, which he established. This organization became one of the most successful voluntary health associations in the United States at that time. It carried on an active health education program, supported vital research on the cause, and later on the prevention of polio. It maintained stocks of respirators for loan to hospitals and gave financial assistance for treatment centers.

Annual fund drives featuring pictures of children who had been crippled as a result of polio were very effective in focusing public attention on this dread disease and in obtaining necessary funds to carry on the Foundation's many programs.

In 1951 and 1952 an epidemic of polio spread across the United States from east to west. It was observed that many cases of mild dysentery preceded the onset of polio by a few weeks. This made it possible to predict the probable occurrence of an outbreak of polio and to prepare for the care of the patients. The spread to the area west of the Rocky Mountains was delayed by the onset of winter. Cases of dysentery began to appear in eastern Oregon the next summer. Fearing an outbreak of polio, the opening of schools was postponed. Public swimming pools were closed. Programs to control mosquitos and flies were increased, and water supplies were thoroughly checked. We tried an experiment in control. In one community, Nyssa, Oregon, a high level of chlorination in the water supply, ("break point chlorination"), was maintained. In nearby communities the usual treatment was carried on. Although it could not be proven that the high level of chlorination accounted for it, the rate of polio infection was considerably less in Nyssa than in the surrounding communities. One other interesting observation on that outbreak of polio was the fact that the community had been prepared to give specialized care to cases. A new hospital had been built in Nyssa, largely in response to a hospital in a neighboring community refusing to admit polio cases out of fear of the disease. The new hospital was designed for isolation and treatment of patients with polio. The hospital had several respirators and had made arrangements to call on the National Foundation for more if needed. Excellent care, of a specialized nature was provided in this moderately rural area.

Isolated cases, small outbreaks, and occasional epidemics continued throughout the country. 1952 was a peak year in the United States with 57,879 reported cases. The CDC maintained a current surveillance of reported cases of polio and published the results. This helped alert health department and physicians in making earlier diagnoses and aided in better community recognition of the disease.

We realized however, that research was the only real hope for control. The means of spread of the viruses had to be found and either an effective preventative, or successful treatment developed. The National Foundation as well as the National Institutes of Health funded many research projects related to polio. In the early thirties the existence of more than one type of polio virus was shown. Then after years of patience and persevering studies a breakthrough occurred in 1949. Dr. John F. Enders, Chief of Virus Research at Children's Hospital in Boston, Massachusetts, demonstrated that the virus could be grown, not only on neurologic tissue, but on other tissues as well. It was determined that initial infection of the gastro-intestinal tract, then invasion of the blood stream, and finally invasion of the brain and spinal cord occurred. Now, the challenge was to develop a safe, effective vaccine. Dr. I. M. Morgan had immunized monkeys with inactivated polio virus in 1948. This was a beginning in the quest for a means of protecting humans. Dr. Enders' discovery was likewise very important in this quest as it was now recognized that a vaccine could be produced using cultured cells to grow the virus.

As a member of the National Polio Foundation's Advisory Committee on Research, I met with Basil O'Conner, the Director of the Foundation (and of the American Red Cross), and other members of the committee during the year 1954. We reviewed applications from Dr. Jonas Salk and Dr. Albert Sabin for funds to continue their research on potential vaccines. Dr. Salk believed in a "killed" vaccine which he hoped would give immunity without causing disease. Dr. Sabin favored an attenuated live virus vaccine. The possible hazard of a live virus vaccine existed in its becoming virulent during production or after inoculation. The Committee recommended support of both researchers.

Dr. Salk was the first to develop a vaccine that was thought to be safe and effective. It had been thoroughly tested in the laboratory and in a limited trial in children. There was no untoward illness in these children, but the effectiveness could not be statistically proven because of the small number of children involved. The vaccine was submitted to the USPHS for testing as to safety. Repeated tests showed that the samples submitted were safe. Approval was given for commercial production. After government testing of samples from many maufacturers the vaccine was released. We were enthusiastic, hoping that at last, polio could be prevented.

The next step was to conduct field trials by vaccinating a much larger group of children. The incidence of poliomyelitis in these children would be compared with the incidence in children who had not received the vaccine. Oregon and California were among the states chosen to be a part of the trial. Careful preparation was made. Vaccines were distributed. The program of administering the vaccine was begun.

Abruptly, however, the program was called to a halt. Totally unexpectedly isolated cases of polio were reported in a few of the inoculated children. Investigation revealed that only those children receiving the vaccine produced by one manufacturer were stricken. Laboratory checks showed that some of the vaccine contained live viruses. How could this have happened? Reasonable precautions had been taken. Investigation revealed that in the manufacture of large quantities of vaccine, a previously unknown phenomena had taken place. Clumping of viruses occasionally occurred. When cultures of the viruses were treated with formalin to kill them, some of the central viruses within the clumps were not killed. Although this occurred infrequently, vaccine containing live viruses was given inadvertently during the trials. This accounted for the cases of polio. Tragically for those thus infected some had residual paralysis and a few children died.

The manufacturing procedure was immediately modified using microfilters to remove any clumps of the virus before treating the cultures with formalin. No further difficulty was encountered, but the appearance of polio in this episode delayed the vaccination program.

Later, Dr. Sabin perfected an attenuated virus oral vacccine. This was given throughout the country starting in 1961. With the cooperation of private physicians, nurses, health department staff, school personnel, the news media, and others, huge numbers of children and adults received sugar cubes containing the oral vaccine. Literally millions of people were vaccinated on "Polio Sundays." Early use of Salk vaccine followed the Sabin vaccine program and brought about spectacular reductions in the number of cases after the 1952 peak. Almost without exception, those that developed polio were persons that had not been protected with the Salk or Sabin vaccines. Not only the safety, but the effectiveness of the vaccines had been proven. There had been concern that persons receiving the live virus vaccine might develop a more virulent virus and spread it to others, particularly to members of their family. This possibility was proven to be almost negligible. Lawrence Schonberger, an epidemiologist with the CDC, discovered that very few such cases occurred each year. There were only seventy-three known endemic vaccine-associated cases in the ten year period, 1969 to 1979. In 1979, only twenty-two cases of polio were reported in the entire United States. Thirteen of these occurred in the Amish epidemic in Pennsylvania, in Iowa, Wisconsin, and in Missouri. Unfortunately, too many individuals have forgotten that there is such a disease. The current hazard results from people who neglect having their children vaccinated and neglect booster vaccinations for themselves. Fear of lawsuits is limiting the number of producers of vaccines and other immunizing agents. A small outbreak could spread before sufficient quantities of vaccine could be produced. Without a known effective treatment, more paralysis and deaths could occur. This must not happen. We must keep up on our vaccination programs to protect our populace.

Research, improved case finding, early supportive treatment, development of effective vaccines to prevent the disease, and education to ensure wide use of the vaccine have been the essential elements in the control of polio. Cooperation of scientists, health departments, voluntary health organizations, physicians, hospitals, and the public has been the key to this success.

INFLUENZA*

Influenza is another disease which has plagued mankind. Although this country has not experienced a pandemic of influenza since the one after World War I, the disease still poses a threat. It is highly communicable. There are many types of the influenza virus and unfortunately new types continue to evolve which may attack millions of people before the populace can be protected by new modified vaccines. World-wide surveillance to recognize and identify new types is our major weapon to minimize this hazard.

The greatest pandemic of influenza in this century, or perhaps of any time in history, occurred in this country in 1918 and 1919. Millions of persons became ill with the disease and hundreds of thousands died. Hardly anyone was able to avoid the virus. Husky men and women, healthy children, teenagers as well as the elderly and debilitated persons were sticken and many succumbed. Persons isolated on ranches and farms, suburban dwellers, and inmates of institutions were not spared. It was easy to understand how persons with the usual contacts in work places, schools, stores, other public places, and within families became infected. How persons or a person isolated on a farm or in a cabin distant from other habitations became infected was a conundrum.

Most cases were treated at home with bed rest, fluids, and aspirin. There were not enough hospitals nor enough doctors and nurses to take care of all of those who became ill. After three to four days, many patients felt better and although physicians warned people to rest for at least a week before getting up, some attempted to return to their former activities after the initial bout of fever. Relapses were common. A massive exudation

*The onset of the disease was sudden, with headache, malaise, sore throat, fever, and chills, loss of appetite, and general aching and weakness. Development of a cough followed.

of fluid took place in the lungs, and people could die, often drowning in their own fluids. Older persons, invalids, and small children were most likely to succumb to the infection, although resolute, strong laborers, unaccustomed to illness and unwilling to stay in bed, frequently died. No one in this country had immunity to this particular virus which ironically, probably was brought back from Europe by returning victorious military personnel.*

Subsequent flu outbreaks due to the influenza virus generally have been milder because most of the new strains of virus are less virulent, the populace has developed some immunity, and because some of the more susceptible groups of the populations have been immunized. Occasional strains which are more virulent, and against which people have little or no immunity and for which vaccines have not been developed, have erupted and spread to various parts of the world including the United States. The Hong Kong flu, swine flu, Russian flu, and Japanese flu are examples.

Vaccines which have proven fairly effective in preventing infection or in minimizing symptoms have been developed. They are recommended for infants, young children, senior citizens, and chronically ill persons who would be most susceptible to the virus and who would be most likely to suffer severe complications or fatal illness. They are also recommended for hospital personnel who would care for influenza patients.

As mentioned, surveillance systems have been established in the United States. One is maintained through the cooperation of the CDC and state health departments. Another world-wide system is maintained under the auspices of the World Health Organization. Health departments of the major nations of the world participate in this surveillance by reporting the incidence of influenza and the type of virus or viruses responsible. New types of influenza are reported and samples of the new virus are transmitted worldwide. This makes it possible to produce more vaccine if required, to incorporate the new virus into vaccines being produced, and to protect the most susceptible persons.

When there is a threat of the spread of more a virulent virus, efforts are made to protect a greater part of the population. The USPHS was criticized for its efforts in having sufficient vaccine produced in 1975 to protect much of the populace against a threatened epidemic of what was thought to be a virulent virus, serologically similar or identical to that of

---

*The virus of that pandemic has not been specifically matched with one of the types or strains known to us today because samples of pharyngeal secretions were not preserved by deep freezing. Techniques for identification were not known then. The electron microscope which made it possible to see viruses was not invented until 1930.

1918. Fortunately, the epidemic did not materialize. Complications from use of the vaccine did occur. Much criticism of the USPHS ensued. What the critics forgot, however, was that if the USPHS had failed to promote the vaccination program and had an epidemic materialized, many lives would have been lost and much illness would have occurred unnecessarily. The same critics who charged "politics", undoubtedly would have criticized the USPHS for not having been prepared!

Although influenza has not been completely eradicated, or controlled, medical science and the application of public health measures have reduced the hazard of epidemics similar to that of 1918-1919. That in itself undoubtedly has saved millions of lives.

4. Health Department Contributions in Control of Sexually Transmitted Diseases

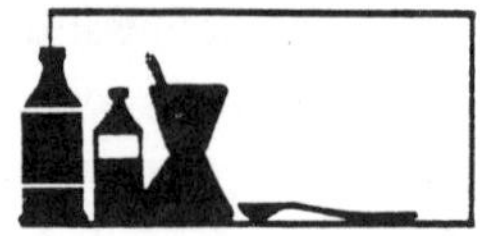

OF ALL THE infectious diseases, those commonly known as STD's have been the most persistent and the most difficult to control. Although treatment of most of these diseases has dramatically improved in recent years, they remain as a serious public health problem. Treatment has progressed from rather ineffective, unproven efforts early in this century to moderately effective, tedious, prolonged treatment and, except for AIDS, on to current, specific, predominantly effective therapy. At this time, a major problem is education of the public to the hazards of STD's, how to avoid them, and in motivating people to apply this knowledge. Case finding and contact investigation are essential.

Until recently, the commonly known STD's were gonorrhea, syphilis, granuloma inguinale, lymphogranuloma venereum, herpes genitalis and chancroid. One form of infectious hepatitis and some of the intestinal infections could be included since they are occasionally transmitted sexually. The recently recognized HIV infection, usually resulting in AIDS, (acquired immune deficiency syndrome), now constitutes a major problem to control and treatment. Although not limited to drug abusers and homosexuals, a majority of cases are found in these groups.

The toll of human life in death, handicaps, sterility, pain and suffering, broken homes, and in the cost of medical care, hospital care, and welfare, taken by these diseases is huge. The control problem is complicated because of promiscuity among both heterosexuals and homosexuals; failure to recognize early symptoms and to seek medical care early; and the continued tendency of the public to stigmatize those who may have contracted an STD. Failure of some physicians to report cases and contacts further complicates the problem.

Although there are as many as twenty-five to thirty STD's many are rare. We will discuss only the most serious and more common. Historically, let us consider syphilis first.*

SYPHILIS

The story of syphilis, often called "lues" in medical circles, is unique among the great plagues in that it was not described until the latter part of the fifteenth century. At that time a dreadful disease called "The Great Pox" swept over the world within a few years. Its origin in Europe is ascribed to the exploratory voyages of Columbus to the West Indies and North America, and the returns of his crew to Spain. The disease was spread throughout Europe by the armies of Spain and France. This infection was no respecter of class. Royalty as well as peasants became victims. There was no effective treatment. The disease was described but it was not differentiated from gonorrhea and other venereal disease, nor were its many forms recognized. It was more virulent at that time than it is today. Many deaths occurred in the early stages of the disease. We can imagine and appreciate the fear that accompanied the spread of this previously unknown disease, which resulted in so many deaths and terrible crippling. The manner of spread was not understood. There was no treatment, nor was there anyway to control it. People were at the disease's mercy.

The first outbreak recognized in this country occurred in Boston, Massachusetts in 1646. It was described in the diary of John Winthrop as "lues venerea". The occurrence involved about sixteen persons, afflicting a sailor, his wife and several babies. The infants became infected as a result of breast feeding from the infected wife. Because Puritanism prevailed, spread of the disease was probably somewhat limited. The disease did crop up in other areas and gradually became more widespread.

When cases were recognized, because there was no specific treatment, special diets, hot baths, fever machines, bleeding, and purging were tried. Mercury rubs were used, but excessive applications often resulted in marked salivation and loss of teeth. William Wallace of Dublin, in 1834, introduced potassium iodide for the treatment of syphilis. It was not until 1837 that Ricord differentiated gonorrhea from syphilis. Between 1875 and 1900, mercury rubs combined with use of potassium-iodide constituted the major

*I present more detail of Syphilis because of the important role of Health Departments in its control, and the parallel to AIDS.

PRIMARY, SECONDARY AND CONGENITAL SYPHILIS
REPORTED CIVILIAN CASES, UNITED STATES
1948–1969

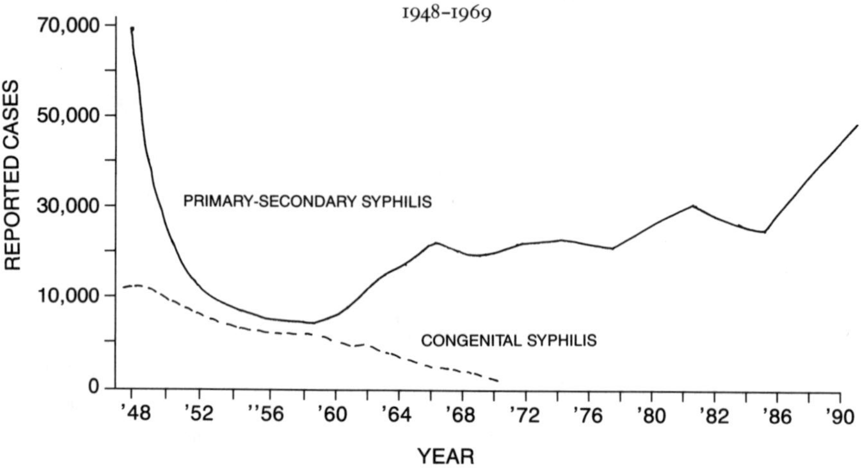

GONORRHEA
REPORTED CIVILIAN CASES, UNITED STATES
1954–1969

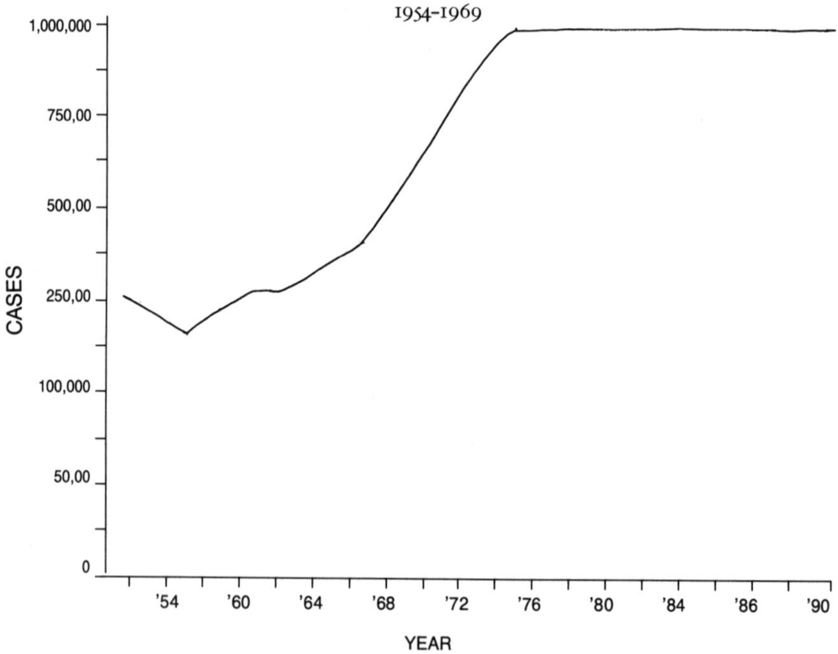

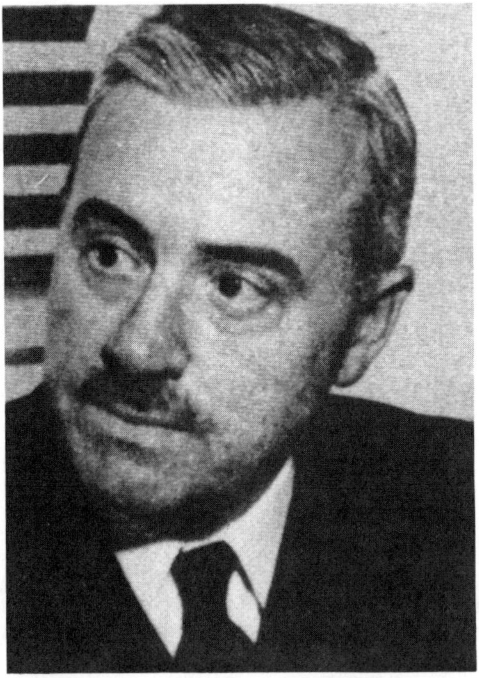

Surgeon General Thomas Parran

treatment. Although this helped to clear some symptoms, it was not a cure. Severe disability and high mortality continued.

In 1874, the American Medical Association became interested, and Dr. S. D. Gross, of Philadelphia, gave the first address on syphilis to the Association in Detroit.

In 1875, Dr. P. H. Bailhache, of the United States Marine Hospital Service, now the USPHS, quite accurately described the disease, its mode of spread, and suggested unsuccessfully, quarantine of infectious cases as was done for smallpox, cholera, yellow fever, and other communicable diseases.

Recognizing the relationship between syphilis and prostitution, the President of the American Medical Association, in 1876, made a plea opposing licensing of prostitution. The Association recommended that city health departments investigate and control cases of syphilis.

At this time some states were becoming concerned about the relationship of brothels to the disease. Although only sporadic enforcement resulted, Virginia in 1877, did enact a law prohibiting brothels. About the same time, some communities in California established Vigilante Committees to drive known prostitutes out of their communities.

Public interest was rising and medical knowledge about the disease began to increase. Neisser, in 1879, discovered the organism causing gonorrhea. This helped clarify some of the symptoms previously attributed to syphilis, and to differentiate the two diseases. Up until this time, attempts to produce the disease in lower animals by inoculation with infectious material had been unsuccessful. In 1903, Metchnikoff, and Roux learned how to inoculate apes and infect them with syphilis. This expanded the possibilities for research a great deal although Philanthropists who were the major source for financing research at that time, were fearful of giving monies for scientific study in such a "shameful" field.

In Germany, in 1905, Fritz Schaudinn, a protozoologist, and Eric Hoffmann, a dermatologist, discovered the corkscrew-shaped bacteria, Spirocheta or Treponema pallidum, which causes syphilis. This was a real breakthrough. About this time, syphilitic infection of the brain resulting in paresis, a mental disorder, and the invasion of the spinal cord, resulting in Tabes dorsalis with a loss of sensation of position of extremities, were recognized as other evidences of the third stage of syphilis.

A few years later, in the twenties, thirties, and forties, physicians realized that much of the serious heart and blood vessel damage that they encountered in patients was due to syphilis.

Another major advance in control was made in 1907 when Wasserman developed the first blood test for syphilis. Named after him, it became one of the essentials in diagnosis and was used as a guide in treatment. Prudery, ignorance of the significance of symptoms, lack of facilities for the diagnosis and treatment, incomplete and unreliable data on the extent of the disease, and fear of ostracism, resulted in continued failure to acknowledge the seriousness of the disease.

The attitude of the public is clearly illustrated in an incident that occurred in 1908. Officers of the USMHS were very much concerned with the large amount of venereal disease occurring in merchant seamen for whose health the Service was responsible. With utmost care they prepared a bulletin for distribution to seamen, explaining the cause, method of spread, and known treatments for the venereal diseases. They particularly made certain that the bulletin would not be offensive. Approval for distribution of the bulletin was requested from the office of the Secretary of the Treasury, George B. Cortelyou. It was returned, "Disapproved", with this note: **"The matter contained in this bulletin is not in keeping with the dignity of the fiscal department of the Government."** As a result of this kind of attitude, ignorance about venereal disease continued unabated.

Because reporting of syphilis was practically non-existent and because deaths from syphilis were almost always attributed to some other cause, either because of failure to diagnose syphilis or to protect the memory of the deceased, or his or her family, true incidence of the disease was not known. When the United States entered World War I in 1917, only nine states had any provision for the reporting of syphilis and in these it was very incomplete. Estimates based on incidence in doctors' offices, clinics for groups such as merchant seamen, studies of patients in mental hospitals, and limited autopsy studies showed that at least 3% to 4% of the total population was infected and that 10% or more of all patients in mental institutions were there because of paresis, or syphilis of the brain. At that time syphilis was more widespread and accounted for more deaths than AIDS does today.

Many scientists throughout the world were searching for a chemical substance that would be effective in treatment. Paul Ehrlich had investigated some 605 chemical compounds for treatment of syphilis without success. What patience! He persisted and on his 606th attempt found an organic arsenical, salvarsan. Ehrlich was first convinced that it would cure a patient with syphilis in one week with one shot. While it did clear up symptoms temporarily, unfortunately they returned. Ehrlich continued his research and on his 914th trial, produced neo-salvarsan.

Salvarsan was called "606". It and neo-salvarsan were made available to the world. Unfortunately, news of their availability and specifics on use were disseminated very slowly. Dr. Thomas Parran commented in his book *Shadow On The Land,* that he was amazed "Ehrlich's discovery of salvarsan in 1910 is news in 1937". These drugs were patented and manufactured only in Germany until World War I. At that time, 1914, exportation of the drugs from Germany was halted. Prices soared to as much as one hundred dollars or more per dose. Dr. Allen McLaughlin, Massachusetts State Health Director, who had initiated a working diagnostic and treatment program for syphilis in his state in 1914, secured state legislation to permit the Massachusetts State Board of Health to produce the drugs. The Board found that the patent descriptions of production were intentionally inaccurately described to prevent manufacture of the drugs by others. Pharmaceutical research soon overcame this obstacle and the drugs were produced and distributed to qualified physicians and clinics. In 1918, several pharmaceutical firms were licensed in the United States to manufacture arsphenamine and neo-arsphenamine.

World War I also resulted in a flurry of interest to control syphilis and other sexually transmitted disease. Congress and the military realized that venereal disease, like shrapnel and bullets, was a serious hazard and could severely incapacitate and handicap military forces. One of every four men suffered from venereal disease in some of the allied armies. On July 9, 1918, Congress established an interdepartmental Social Hygiene Board. The secretaries of War, Navy, and the Treasury were members. A division of Venereal Disease Control was established in the USPHS.

One million dollars, currently equivalent in purchasing power to about fifteen million dollars, was appropriated for grants to states to establish Venereal Disease Control Programs meeting federal standards. Within one year, forty-six of the then forty-eight states cooperated. Clinics and public health laboratories were established. Drugs were provided for those who could not afford to pay for treatment. Mandatory reporting of syphilis was one of the requirements. Limited educational programs were established. Secretary of the Treasury, William G. McAdoo, sponsored a bill for a national program of syphilis control. As Director General of the Railways, he had placards posted in Pullman washrooms, industrial plants, and other public places warning of the hazards of venereal disease and urging treatment. This was in marked contrast to earlier attitudes. General John J. Pershing issued what was considered to be the most notable health order in Military history, the famous G.O.N.T.T., which put all house of prostitution out of bounds of military personnel. The American Red Cross established VD treatment clinics around military camps.

Public enthusiasm for any measure to help end the war, terminated abruptly with the cessation of fighting. The Roaring Twenties were on. Syphilis was soon forgotten and in fact, was again hidden from public view. Appropriations for VD control were radically reduced in 1920, and they were completely abolished by the Congress in 1926. Fortunately some states had become aware of the seriousness of the problem and continued limited programs to control syphilis.

The Great Depression, beginning with the stock market crash of 1929, halted financing of most of these venereal disease control programs. Apathy, and general lack of public awareness of the serious hazards of syphilis, prevented any real control measures. The cause of the disease and the method of spread were known. Fairly reliable diagnostic tests were available. Although it was lengthy, lasting a minimum of eighteen months, a specific treatment was available.

This was the situation when I first became acquainted with the problem of syphilis. I can remember my introduction to education about the disease in 1926, as a pre-med student at the University of Washington. All male students were required to attend a special health program in Meany Hall. A description of syphilis was given and slides were shown depicting the various symptoms and stages of the disease, including pictures of the primary chancre, secondary rash, and finally, of advanced cases with bone deformities, large areas of ulceration, and patients with brain involvement, nerve damage, and heart impairment. It was a shocking presentation which caused some students to faint and be carried out of the auditorium.

My next involvement was seeing clinical cases of syphilis in medical school. There were hundreds of people coming to the clinic for diagnosis and treatment of the disease. I vividly remember patients with saddle noses, the bridge of the nose having been destroyed. Some were blind, deaf, or both, often from congenital syphilis, (some with characteristic Hutchinson's, or notched teeth). Other patients had "Tabes", (those who had lost sensation in feet and legs and who clopped along not knowing where their feet were). If these patients closed their eyes, they lost their balance and fell. Other patients had huge ulcers on their legs or other parts of their bodies. Some had heart conditions, huge aneurysms, (enlargement of major arteries), gummas or syphilitic areas of destruction of vital organs of the body. Occasionally we saw persons with primary chancre or ulcer of the sexual organs or with a generalized rash characteristic of the secondary stage. We also occasionally saw an early case of paresis, usually a person with delusions of grandeur. They were the ones who often said, although obviously poor, that they were wealthy and claimed to own farms, ranches, apartment buildings, estates, and yachts. We saw infants and small children who had received the infection from their mothers during pregnancy. Syphilis was the "Great Imitator". Diagnosis was often complicated and syphilis, or lues, could not be ruled out until the results of the Wasserman test, or "dark field"* were known.

There are three stages of syphilis, between which a patient may appear to be completely normal. The primary manifestation of infection is the chancre. Spread of the spirochete, causing the disease, is usually from an infected mucous surface of one person to another, commonly during intercourse. Within a month a small papule, or pimple, develops at the site of infection. It becomes a small ulcer with a pearly hard ring crown. generally there is only one chancre. Darkfield microscopic examination of smears from the chancre often reveals the spirochetes. With or without treatment, the chancre heals and disappears. Unless the individual has been diagnosed and adequately treated, this is merely a lull in the visible evidence of invasion of the body by the spirochetes.

*Microscopic examination for spirochetes (special illumination).

Generally about two to three months after the appearance of the chancre, the spirochetes have spread throughout a great part of the body. A skin rash appears and lesions of the mucous membranes, varying from small papules to ulceration, so-called "mucous patches", may occur on any of the mucous areas of the body. These lesions usually are teeming with spirochetes. Diagnostic blood tests are almost always positive during this stage. Again, the superficial lesions of this second phase of the disease heal spontaneously even though a diagnosis may not have been made and adequate treatment given. As previously stated, this is merely a lull in symptoms while the spirochetes consolidate in various organs and prepare for major destruction.

If adequate treatment has not been given, the tertiary stage, after a period of freedom from symptoms ensues, usually within two to three years. It may be delayed for as long as eight to ten years. Destruction of almost any part of the body may then occur. Most of the patients were relatively young, varying in age from thirty to the mid-fifties. One cannot help but see the similarities of this disease to infection with HIV and AIDS.

The most pitiful cases were those in babies and small children.* Once diagnosis of syphilis was made, we had to explain to the patient, or the parents of a child, the necessity for eighteen months of treatment. To come to the clinic every week for a year and a half was a great burden for the patient, but many of them, recognizing the hazard of incomplete treatment, did come.

I am afraid that as students we were unaware of the public health implications of the disease. We knew of the communicability of many of the new patients with lesions, and we did take precautions to protect ourselves. We were not told to report the cases to the health department. I doubt if the record clerks reported these cases either. We did not check on other than immediate family contacts. Generally, we were too busy diagnosing and treating patients to appreciate the importance of control and to find out where the patients may have been infected. In the advanced type of cases that we chiefly saw, determination of the source of infection would have been difficult. From time to time a patient with a primary chancre, a secondary rash, or a positive Wasserman test would

*Babies often born prematurely, usually had snuffies, mucous patches, an intractable diaper rash, and cranial bossing (rounded protuberances). The baby was commonly stunted. Some claimed that these babies looked like "little, dried-up old men". Often they had anemia and jaundice. If the child lived, it often had convulsions, was mentally retarded, and frequently developed blindness and deafness. The incisor teeth were notched. Later in life many developed sabre shins and saddle noses. Blood and spinal tests were used to confirm the diagnosis.

express real concern and would ask what they could tell their marital partner. They realized as we did, that acquiring the infection extra-maritally could be the basis for the break-up of the family. We did explain measures they could take to protect their partners. (Lawsuits were not common then.)

After graduation from medical school, and as a county health officer in two small counties in Oregon, I conducted weekly VD Clinics in which I treated many individuals who had acquired syphilis. The patients were very appreciative and usually returned on schedule for their treatments. It was very gratifying to see large ulcers, often they were deep and huge, or other evidence of syphilis clear up. Those fortunate enough to come in early in the course of their disease and who completed the recomended treatment had an excellent chance of a complete cure. Congenital cases and those with tertiary symptoms could only look forward to an arrest of the disease.

Screening of the population for syphilis was limited. Some states, Oregon and California included, had laws requiring pre-marital blood testing for syphilis. Most hospitals included the Wasserman test in the admittance exam. About 4% of individuals tested were found to have syphilis. Unfortunately, many young people would not wait the three days required for testing and got married in a neighboring state where the testing was not required. I have seen many cases of syphilis that could have been detected years earlier if pre-marital couples had not circumvented the law.

In 1937, in establishing a new health program in Wasco and Sherman counties in Oregon, one small city adopted an ordinance requiring all food service personnel to have examinations for tuberculosis, other communicable disease, and to have a blood test for syphilis. Many criticized the blood testing portion of the program as unnecessary, pointing out that syphilis was not transmitted through food service. In reality, more than twice as much syphilis was found in these exams than was found in pre-marital examinations. Those found with positive tests sought treatment and with continued treatment, were permitted to engage n food service since they were not infectious.

Contacts were checked. There were three houses of prostitution in The Dalles. Each had a madam and three or four girls. Prior to establishment of the health department in 1937, the police had required the girls to obtain cards from private physicians certifying to their freedom from venereal disease. The intent was good but the girls used the the cards to assure patrons of their freedom from disease. In actuality, no physician could certify that a girl, after her first sexual contact following a careful examination and laboratory testing, would be free of the spirochete or other venereal disease organisms. I met with the police chief and the doctors and explained the hazard. The practice of issuing cards was stopped.

As our Venereal Disease Clinic became better known through word of mouth, we had young people coming to us with primary and secondary syphilis and gonorrhea. We obtained names of contacts, and did check on them. In many instances we found that a girl in one of the houses was named as a source. We immediately called her in; gave her a thorough examination including smears and blood test, and checked her to see if she had any suspicious signs of infection. If she was found to be infected we referred her to her own physician for treatment, or we instituted treatment. We attempted to have the houses closed, but at that time, they were too well-accepted by the public. In fact, many people thought that the houses were essential in the community. On examining some of the girls named as contacts I learned that many were previously married women with a child or children to support.

With the establishment of many new local health departments in 1937-38, this type of control was markedly increased.

Public education regarding the STD's however, was almost non-existent in 1935. The words syphilis, gonorrhea, and venereal disease were still taboo. Newspapers generally would not use the words for fear of offending their readers. I do not remember seeing any newspaper or magazine articles, or even references to these subjects, until Dr. Thomas Parran, Surgeon General of the USPHS exposed the seriousness of the problem in his book, *Shadow on the Land*.

Dr. Parran, as a member of a commission of doctors, had visited the Scandinavian countries to determine whether their claims of success in the control of syphilis were warranted and if so, to learn how they made such great progress as compared to ours. The Commission found that the claims had not been exaggerated. The Danish program dated back 150 years. Ninety-three percent of all known cases completed a full course of treatment. Most everyone in Denmark was well-informed about the disease and there was no hesitation on the part of the press or the public to discuss syphilis as a disease. Success of the program was the result of public health control measures. It was not based on a social difference from that of the United States, since gonorrhea was just as prevalent in Denmark as it was in this country.

Similar programs were being conducted in Great Britain, Norway, and Sweden, and in these countries, too, control of the disease was far superior to ours.

Dr. Parran pointed out that in the United States, in 1935, the newspapers and magazines thought it improper to use the word syphilis. Wasserman tests were done only sporadically in hospitals. Many hospitals would not admit known cases of syphilis and very few hospital beds were set aside for care of such persons. Only one half the number of Wasserman tests were performed in the United States on a per capita basis as were done in Denmark, although the need for such screening was far greater in the United States. Twenty to forty percent of patients in this country dropped out of treatment before they had completed even twenty of the seventy-five doses needed.

Dr. Parran further pointed out that ten percent of all insanity and fifteen percent of all blindness in this country was due to syphilis. Ten to twelve percent of all the deaths from heart disease were attributable to syphilis. Surveys showed that three to four million people in the United States were infected. Dr. Parran performed Kahn tests, (an improved blood test for syphilis), on a number of domestics in Washington D.C., and found fifty percent of them to be positive. What an outcry for action there would have been if these had been cases of smallpox, diphtheria, or polio. There were very few clinics or local programs to combat the disease and relatively little was being done by state health departments.

In Washington, one physician reported that he sent reports of cases of syphilis to the local health department. After a time, a secretary from the department called and told him not to send any more of these reports as the department did not have the staff to follow up on the cases. The reports were merely cluttering up her desk. Congress and state legislatures apparently were not interested in appropriating funds to diagnose and treat this "hush-hush" disease. Our government spent $264 million to control tuberculosis in cattle between 1917 and 1935. During the same period, $8 million were appropriated for the control of syphilis. Again, one wonders about our priorities!

The lack of interest was not limited to congress and state legislatures. In Montana, the state legislature in 1935, enacted, and the Governor duly signed, what was termed a Gin Marriage Law. It provided for a three-day waiting period and a medical examination of all marriage applicants. There was a great public reaction against the new law. Within months, the people voted the law out.

In addition to meager appropriations for control programs, laboratory services were very scarce and many of those doing blood tests for syphilis were not competent. Nine states limited diagnostic tests for syphilis to the indigent although they provided unlimited free tests for tuberculosis. Dr. Parran was determined to overcome this apathy.

To emphasize the means of spread of syphilis, Dr. Parran told of a series of cases found, following the performances of a traveling show. In an eastern seaboard state one of the performers, Little Eva, had sold her personal favors after the show. These had proven to be very popular, but many of those who had accepted the favors paid for them dearly by acquiring syphilis. In another instance, a popular eighteen year old high school senior with sores on his month was responsible for seventeen cases of syphilis; the origin being his kisses.

Dr. Parran made many talks to important organizations. He presented the facts to congress and proposed a program for control. He wrote his excellent book on syphilis previously referred to. He was actively supported by the American Social Hygiene Association. That Association published and widely distributed the book in 1937. This was the first real breakthrough into the media. He suggested a platform for action. *First,* find every case of syphilis early. In addition to the physician performing a Wasserman test on his or her patient whenever there was the slightest suspicion of any lesion being due to a syphilitic infection, he recommended the test as part of every medical examination. He suggested that these tests be made on all patients admitted to a hospital and particularly on all obstetrical patients. He proposed that every applicant for life insurance, all applicants for a marriage license, and all law breakers receive Wasserman tests. He suggested screening all new employees in industry. *Second,* Dr. Parran proposed that every case of syphilis be reported to the health department to assure follow-up and investigation of contacts. He emphasized that confidentiality of records of patients must be strictly maintained. *Third,* every patient should be assured of complete treatment with a cure, if possible, but certainly enough to make the patient non-infectious. He recommended appropriations of public funds to provide clinic facilities, trained public health personnel, laboratory services, and the necessary drugs for the program. He particularly emphasized the need for team work, for the fullest cooperation between the private physician, medical societies, the American Social Hygiene Association, government, health departments, and the general public.

Dr. Parran's efforts brought results. The most significant development was the acceptance by the press of syphilis as a problem, and of the need to present it to their readers as a disease. People became aware of it, and we, as health officers, spoke out about the problem and the need for funds to deal with it without fear of being criticized or of offending the public.

Congress initially appropriated $8 million for venereal disease control, 3 million dollars for maternal and child health programs, and several million to aid states in establishing local health departments and community venereal disease control programs. This was a beginning. Appropriations were increased modestly and continued. Health programs emphasizing venereal disease control were expanded throughout the country. Again, World War ii, 1941-45, curtailed the development of all these programs.

During World War II, The American Social Hygiene Association made surveys of houses of prostitution and made reports on the results to military and state and local health officials. The military requested closing of the houses and put them off limits. It took considerable time, effort, and pressure to close all of them due to objections of some business men having a financial interest in the buildings used, of police officials who really believed that sex-related crimes would increase if the houses were closed, and of special interest groups. Actually, it was found that sex-related crimes decreased when the houses were closed. I remember a prediction of a Canadian health officer, made in a talk in Oregon outlining success in reducing incidences of syphilis and gonorrhea in Canada. He told us that local special interests had publicized a probable increase of attacks on wives and daughters by sex maniacs, the driving of prostitutes out of cities into suburban communities, loss of control, and an increase in general crime. He stated that none of these predictions materialized. Just as anticipated, on the front page of the Oregon newspapers parallel columns appeared, one quoting police officials and businessmen making predictions of dire results if the houses were closed, and the other quoting the Canadian Health Officer, refuting the predictions based on actual experience. Eventually, the large majority of the houses were closed with the support of the military. Without the latter, I doubt that it could have been accomplished.

As State Health Officer in Oregon, I received the American Social Hygiene reports and learned that houses of prostitution were still operating in The Dalles, Pendleton, and Klamath Falls, Oregon. This was in the early forties. houses were accepted as a way of life and considered to be an essential element in these rugged western communities. As former health officer in The Dalles, I personally visited the community, talked with the mayor and city councilmen, and was assured that the houses would be closed. I insisted on visiting the houses with the police chief. We saw each madam in the three houses, explained that they must be closed, and then we actually padlocked the doors of the establishments. I remember one of the madams patting the chief on the shoulder and saying, "I told you that this was coming chief. I knew we would have to close up." The houses were closed and the incidence of venereal disease did drop.

The major reason for the decline in cases from this source is one of simple arithmetic. It was recognized that many of these prostitutes or hookers would continue their activities on an individual basis as would bar girls, pick ups and others. On their own, if infected, one of these girls could spread the infection to two or three men in one evening. In an organized house of prostitution the same girl could potentially infect as many as fifty or more. With fifteen to twenty times as many contacts the chances of the girl becoming infected, if she had previously not been, and of spreading infection were increased tremendously.

The military continued to receive reports through the fifties, sixties, and seventies on sources of infection in military personnel. When a specific bar or night spot was found to be a frequent site of pick-ups, that establishment was placed out of bounds until policies changed. This proved effective.

With routine blood testing on pre-natal, and pre-marital persons, on all hospital admissions, and frequently occupants of jails, prisons, and institutions, and as part of pre-employment exams, case-finding improved. Private physicians took more interest in diagnosing and treating the disease. In addition, patients were diagnosed and treated in health department clinics. Special facilities were established in many states for the treatment of babies and small children with congenital syphilis.

Up until this time the major problem in control had been the length of time required for treatment and the difficulty in keeping patients on treatment and under surveillance for eighteen months. In 1938, a dramatic breakthrough occurred. In 1928, Sir Alexander Fleming had discovered a mold, penicillin, that destroyed many bacteria. His very significant discovery was overlooked for many years, until Sir Howard Walter Foley led a team that purified penicillin, making its use possible in humans. Beginning in 1938, knowledge of its value in combatting bacterial infections began to spread. The benefits of penicillin in treatment of syphilis became apparent. Patients with syphilis now received treatment for days instead of months. Initially, penicillin was given intramuscularly for seven days or more. Then preparations were developed that were effective in treating early and secondary cases with only one, and at most, two shots. With this improvement in treatment and better case-finding the incidence of syphilis dropped dramatically. By 1950, cases of tertiary syphilis, tabes, and paresis were rarities. Today, paresis as a cause of mental disease is practically unknown.

Case-finding has been an important factor in curbing the infection. When health departments learned of cases they interviewed patients, generally determined the names of the contacts and arranged either for the contacts to see their own physician, or to visit a health department clinic for examination. Specially trained interviewers became very skilled in explaining the benefits of reaching all contacts and in obtaining the patients cooperation in locating them. Appreciating the importance of contact investigation and the skill of these interviewers, some private physicians have utilized their service. The importance and value of finding all contacts on a strictly confidential basis is illustrated by an incident that occurred in southern California in the early seventies.

A young woman came into a health clinic in Riverside, California. She had a generalized rash and a few mucous patches. Examination and blood testing revealed that she had secondary syphilis. She explained that she was a waitress in a small restaurant at a truck stop in a neighboring county. She was queried about contacts. When the need to find them for diagnosis and treatment was explained to her, the patient produced a "little black book" in which she had truck license numbers and names of the drivers who might have been exposed. With the cooperation of the CDC and a number of state and local health departments, over 150 contacts through out the country were checked and at least fourteen previously unknown cases of syphilis were found. This not only illustrates the value of learning of contacts and checking up on them, but serves to demonstrate how one individual can spread the disease, inadvertently, across boundaries to involve people in many states. Adequately staffed health departments are essential for this kind of control.

With enlightenment of the public, good case-finding, and modern rapid treatment, the incidence of the disease has been reduced so much that an insufficient number of new cases of syphilis were found to justify pre-marital and other well-person testing. Only because of the need to prevent congenital syphilis and out of concern for the expectant mother has pre-natal testing been continued.

Dr. Parran's vision of complete control of syphilis within one generation has not been fully achieved, but within two generations his "Plan For Control" has been successful. Although changes in attitudes toward sex and sex practices have promoted the spread of all STD's, syphilis is still far less common than many of the other STD's.

It is unfortunate that we do not have sufficient health department staffs and authorization from government to carry on the same kind of control program for HIV infection.

GONORRHEA*

One of the most prevalent of the sexually transmitted diseases in the United States today is gonorrhea, (GC). It is estimated currently that there are 2.5-3 million cases occurring each year in this country. As I mentioned in the discussion on syphilis, Neisser discovered the bacterium, Neisseria gonorrhea, in 1879, and gonorrhea was recognized as a separate disease. Its relationship to brothels, known in France as "clapier", probably accounts for the slang expression designating gonorrhea as a "dose of clap."

In males, the symptoms are rather painful. Infants' eyes may be infected during passage through an infected birth canal. Women may be suffering from the disease without recognizable symptoms.** The female with a chronic infection, often without recognized symptoms, is the greatest proliferator of the disease.

Until the late thirties there was no specific treatment for gonorrhea. I remember the treatment which we gave to patients in the medical school

---

*A few days after exposure to an infected person, the exposed individual notices an intense burning sensation and considerable pain on urination. This is as a result of inflammation of the uretha, the tubal passage in the penis. A purulent (pus-like) discharge generally accompanies the inflammation. The infection can spread to the prostate gland, testes, and epididymis. Occasionally it invades the bladder and sometimes the bloodstream. The latter can result in involvement of the heart, joints, and the brain. The pharynx and the rectum can also be infected. Spread by the hands, can result in infection of the eye which if untreated can lead to blindness.

*They may have urethritis with the discomfort on urination and frequency. Complications often occur with infection of the Fallopian tubes, ovaries, and occasionally surrounding tissues resulting in pelvic infiammatory disease, PID. More generalized symptoms with fever and malaise result. The heart, brain, joints, rectum, bladder, and eyes may all be attacked just as they may be in the male. Gonorrhea is the most common cause of sterility in females. This results from scarring and obliterating strictures in the Fallopian tubes.

clinics. We encouraged them to force fluids, get plenty of rest, maintain a good diet, and to refrain from drinking alcohol and from having intercourse. We often prescribed alternative weeks of taking sodium bicarbonate for one week followed by taking a weak acid-reacting drug, methenamine, for a week. This treatment was of some value. A few of our male patients developed partial strictures of the urethra. Under supervision we passed urethral sounds, a metallic type probe, to stretch the urethra, and break up scar tissue strictures, and pockets of inflammation. This was a very painful procedure for the patients as it was done without benefit of an anesthetic. Those that developed inflammation of the prostrate required massage of the prostrate. Passing of sounds and massage of the prostrate was required twice a week.

Those men with generalized symptoms and women with pelvic inflammatory disease (PID), or other major complications were usually hospitalized with complete bed rest, sedatives, and the forcing of fluids, often intravenously or subcutaneously. Patients generally recovered but often it took weeks of therapy. Until about 1900, babies born to mothers with gonorrhea commonly developed eye infections resulting in blindness. This was due to exposure to the bacteria during the birth process. It was discovered that an instillation of weak silver nitrate solution in the eyes immediately after birth generally prevented the development of gonorrheal ophthalmitis, or infection of the eye. In the early 1900's most state health departments where they had been established, adopted regulations requiring the instillation of 1% silver nitrate solution drops in the eyes of all newborn babies immediately after birth. Today, some states permit the substitution of antibiotics. This dramatically reduced the incidence of blindness in infants as the result of infection with gonorrhea. A significant amount of blindness is still caused by this disease.

Fortunately, most patients recover from an attack of gonorrhea. I remember as an assistant county physician in Portland, Oregon, I had responsibility for medical care of the Multnomah County Jail inmates. Some of the prisoners were infected with gonorrhea. We isolated them, explained the disease and the hazard of spread, and outlined a conservative treatment program. They did get rest—there was not much else to do in jail. Most of them forced fluids—alcohol was not available—and they did alternate baking soda and methenamine as prescribed. These patients did exceedingly well on this regime and very few developed complications. In fact, they did better than many of the patients coming to our medical school clinics!

No real change in the care or treatment of patients occurred until the late thirties when sulphanilamide therapy was introduced. This was very effective, requiring only one or two weeks of treatment. Even those individuals who had developed complications responded quite well to sulphonamide therapy. There were recurrences and many reinfections, a major problem, but the incidence of complications was markedly reduced. The next advance in treatment came with the introduction of penicillin. One injection of slow absorbing penicillin G. given with a drug called probenecid, oral antibiotics, usually resulted in a cure.

With such effective treatment, many expected that gonorrhea would soon be controlled. I have heard young people say, "What? A dose of 'clap'? That's nothing. Not as bad as a cold!" Major problems remained, however. These included promiscuity, dissemination of the disease by girls and women who were unaware of their infection, and drug resistance of new strains of the organism causing the disease. Re-infection was a recurring problem, and a frustrating one. Contact investigation was more difficult than with syphilis because of patients misconceptions that GC was not as serious a disease. Shortage of health department staffs and deficiencies in reporting limit control.

To combat the resistant strains, new treatment schedules have been developed which, if followed, provide about a 95% cure of patients. Close supervision is required by medical personnel to insure cure and freedom form other venereal disease or conditions which may have been acquired with the gonorrheal infection. Some of the most pitiful cases that we see in the VD Clinics today are the girls, some of them as young as twelve years, who not only have contracted gonorrhea, syphilis, or HIV infection, but who, in addition, are pregnant. These require not only a great deal of skill in treatment, but also in handling social complications. Another problem that confronts us in control is the failure of a patient who has had gonorrhea to develop immunity to the disease. We do not have a vaccine to prevent it. As stated, individuals can and do suffer repeated infections, some many times. Better communication with the patient and good explanations, both of the hazards of repeated infections, and of acquiring other STD's such as "AIDS", and the means of avoiding them seems to be the only solution. In the meantime, until a vaccine is developed, gonorrhea continues to be a significant public health problem.

CHLAMYDIA
LYMPHGRANULOMA VENEREUM

This is one of the recognized venereal diseases that is caused by inclusion bodies growing only in cells. It was first described in France in 1913. The disease is common throughout the United States afflicting four or more million men and women. If it is not treated early, it can be very serious, resulting in severe disability and requiring hospitalization and surgery to relieve strictures.* Diagnosis, particularly in the early stages of the disease, may be difficult. A skin test, known as the Frei Test, cell cultures, complement-fixation tests, and blood tests, are helpful. Treatment for early cases utilizing antibiotics, tetracycline, and chloramphenicol, has been found to be effective.

The disease occurs worldwide, and unfortunately, appears to be increasing.

HERPES GENITALIS**

This is another venereal disease caused by a virus, herpes virus type II. It was first recognized in the latter part of this century. It too, seems to be increasing and probably is now a greater problem than syphilis. It is estimated that as many as thirty million Americans are infected. It is more common in those failing to maintain the best personal hygiene. The disease is most serious in women. Some researchers have implicated it with cervical cancer. It is particularly serious in pregnant women. often resulting in miscarriage, stillbirth, or in an infected, retarded child. At term, in a known case, a Caesarian section delivery is usually opted for to avoid infection of the baby. A simple skin test for the herpes virus in those having symptoms of the disease, aids in diagnosis. As there is no known cure, only supportive treatment can be given.

---

*A constriction or shutting off of a tube e.g. outlet of bladder.

**Patients often have localized pain, genital lesions, small pimples becoming blisters, enlarged lymph glands, and may have generalized symptoms of fever and malaise. Stress aggravates the condition. Symptomatic treatment with drugs, acyclor and vaccines, is partially successful, depending on the extent of the disease. Relapses of symptoms constitute the greatest problem as the virus continues to survive in the body.

CHANCROID*

This disease, also called soft chancre, is a more common sexually transmitted disease than lymphogranuloma venereum. It, too, occurs worldwide and is more prevalent in the southern part of the United States than in the rest of the country. It was found to be due to an infection with a bacterium, a gram negative bacillus named Hemophilus ducreyi. Diagnosis is primarily made based on the case history and symptoms. Use of a skin test with discovery of the bacillus confirm the diagnosis. Treatment with antibiotics for one to two weeks can be successful. Untreated, the disease is usually self-limiting.

GRANULOMA INGUINALE**

This is another of the venereal diseases which, fortunately, is somewhat rare in this country. It is a lingering, chronic, relapsing type of infection causing deep ulceration of the skin and of the ano-genital areas. It is caused by a bacteria, Donovania granulomatis, which form the so-called Donovan bodies within the tissue cells. Fortunately many persons seem to have a natural resistance to this disease as all of those exposed do not contract it. Often a marital partner of a known case will not become infected.

Those who do contract the disease have little resistance to it and usually do not develop resistance. The disease may last for many years. Before antibiotics, antimony compounds were used in treatment. Now use of the newer antibiotics can be successful when given early.

HEPATITIS B

As mentioned earlier, Hepatitis B and some of the enteric diseases such as amoebic dysentery, may occasionally be transmitted through sexual acts.

---

*Three to ten days after exposure, a small lesion appears at the site of the invasion. Ulceration occurs and the inguinal glands, usually on one side only, enlarge to form buboes, similar to those occurring in lymphogranuloma venereum. These may soften and rupture. Fever, chills, and general malaise usually accompany the lymph node involvement.

**About four to twelve weeks after exposure rather painless nodules appear on the skin or mucous membranes of the genital, perineal, and inguinal areas. These ulcerate, spread, and may involve large areas of the lower body; spreading onto the abdomen and even to the thighs. Healing and scarring may occur on one border of a lesion and spread on another border. Often secondary infection occurs with advanced infection. Treatment becomes even more difficult.

Hepatitis B has become a major problem accounting for more deaths than AIDS! Transmission through blood transfusions and to medical personnel through accidental contact with contaminated blood has occurred in the past. An effective vaccine is now available. It should be used to protect health personnel most likely to be exposed to cases, freqent travellers, drug abusers, patients with AIDS, and debilitated persons. Because of its present hight cost, it is not recommended for all persons, but only those at greatest risk.*

AIDS
HIV INFECTION

The mere mention of AIDS induces fear in many people. Articles related to it are found almost daily in the press, while comments on the subject are heard relentlessly on radio and television. The confounding fact about this disease, is that AIDS, Acquired Immune Deficiency Syndrome, was unknown or at least unrecognized in the United States until 1981. It was then that Dr. Michael Gottlieb, a medical researcher, clinician, and teacher at the University of California, Los Angeles, first observed three patients with severe immune suppression and unusual infections. He studied these cases thoroughly, not only doing complete physical examinations and taking detailed histories, but also by applying all of the laboratory tests that might be helpful in diagnosis. These examinations only showed that this disease was different from any that Dr. Gottlieb had ever seen before.

Because they were so different, he reported the cases in June, 1981. He called the condition Acquired Immune Deficiency Syndrome, AIDS. Soon other physicians, primarily in San Francisco and New York, were reporting similar cases that they were observing. The first of these seemed to be predominantly in drug abusers in New York and in homosexuals in the San Francisco area. In Los Angeles, it seemed to be occurring in both drug abusers and homosexuals. No known treatment was effective for these patients. ALL soon died. As the number of case reports of AIDS increased, it was recognized that a devastating epidemic was developing in homosexual and drug abuser groups. By 1987, over twenty thousand

*Before discussing AIDS, we should mention one more STD, genital warts, because it is thought to afflict two or three million Americans each year. Symptoms are usually mild with warts appearing around the genitalia, one or two months after sexual exposure to an infected individual. The infection is due to one of many viruses. It is usually self-limited.

cases had been reported, and some estimated that as many as a million persons had been infected with the HIV (1) virus. Of these, many had quiescent, or latent infections. Others had unrecognized AIDS that had not been reported. It was accurately predicted that there could be as many as one-quarter million cases of AIDS reported in the United States by 1990. Now the disease had become pandemic.

In 1983, physicians in France discovered the virus responsible for AIDS. They designated it as the lymphadenopathy associated virus, or LAV (a retro virus). About the same time, Robert C. Gallo, M.D., Chief of the Laboratory of Tumor Cell Biology, National Cancer Institute, found the retrovirus in AIDS patients in the United States. He designated the virus as Human T Cell Lymphovirus, Type III. It is now referred to as HIV(1)*. It was found to be a very minute virus, smaller than most viruses. It was somewhat similar to a virus found in Iceland, in sheep having visna, an unusually fatal disease involving the nervous system of the sheep. The disease had been eradicated in Iceland. AIDS has also been recognized in epidemic form in Africa and Haiti.

Where did the virus resulting in AIDS come from? Was it the result of a mutation or change in form of similar viruses? Was it imported from Africa, or the flocks of sheep of Iceland, from France, Haiti, or other parts of the world? It is now believed that the infection originated in Africa.

Introduction of the virus into the United States probably was by an infected visitor to a club on Long Island, New York. Although initially the HIV was found primarily in drug abusers and homosexuals, a few cases were discovered in individuals infected after having received blood transfusions or blood products prior to March, 1985. At that time a program to test all potential blood donors for antibodies to the virus was initiated and those testing positive were rejected. I would emphasize that the hazard of infection with HIV through the blood donor program has been largely eliminated as the result of rigid blood testing in donors, both for HIV(1) and HIV(2).

Before discussing further how the virus of AIDS is spread, let us consider the course of the infection and the various forms it may assume. Once infected, either through infected blood or semen, the virus spreads rapidly through the body. The virus must be enclosed in a blood cell, primarily a T-lymphocyte or a helper cell, if it is to survive. It often invades cells

---

*An HIV(2), although rare, is now being found in the U.S.A.

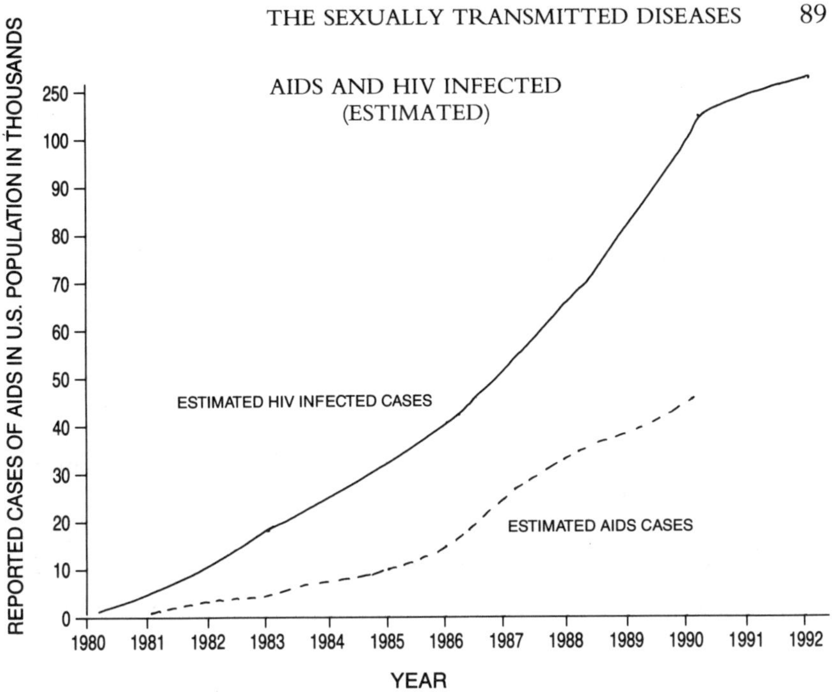

of the central nervous system. Fortunately, the necessity of enclosure in a blood cell limits transmission of the disease to direct contact.

During the next six to eight weeks it attacks the immune system of the individual, particularly the T-4, CD4+ helper cells and another lymphocyte, the B-cell, which produces antibodies. The body attempts to destroy the virus and in this attempt develops some antibodies to the virus. For reasons unknown, the antibodies are not effective. They do however, make possible the recognition of the presence of the virus when the blood is tested for the antibodies. The available tests include the ELISA, enzyme linked immune sorbene assay, the Western Blot test, and the IFA, immune fluorescence antibody test. The ELISA is designed to be especially sensitive to the antibodies. Because of this, the test may occasionally give what is termed a false positive. The only infection that the test might miss is the very early infection in which an individual has not yet developed antibodies. It is thought that such an oversight rarely occurs, perhaps once in a million or more tests.

The Western Blot test on the other hand, is not as sensitive. It identifies antibodies to proteins of specific molecular weight. This test would miss occasional cases because of this specificity. Only about 75% of individuals having a positive ELISA test, test positive with the Western Blot test. If the latter is positive, one can be very certain that the blood is from an individual infected with the HIV. The IFA test is being found to correlate very well with the clinical findings of individuals having the infection. When used together, these tests complement each other and are very accurate.

A new screening test which takes only a few minutes to perform has been approved by the Food and Drug Administration. It is the Recombigen HIV-Latex Agglutination Test. The SUDS test, single use diagnostic system, is a simple color test using only a drop of blood which can be obtained from a finger prick. It is inexpensive. Its results however, are not definitive. They must be confirmed by other tests.

The course of infection with the HIV(1) can vary considerably in different individuals depending on their general health, diet, mode of living, use of tobacco, alcohol, and harmful drugs, sexual practices, and other factors that influence ones health.

During the periods of invasion and attack of the immune system, an individual may experience fatigue and fever. Some individuals have diarrhea and swelling of lymph glands of the groin, neck, or armpits. Symptoms may simulate those of infectious mononucleosis. Many persons infected with the virus may not have any symptoms during this initial period of invasion. Following this phase the infection may become latent, somewhat similar to the latent periods occurring in patients with syphilis.

In both of these infections, one with HIV, and the other with the spirochete, the only evidence during the periods of latency may be the positive blood test and changes in the lymphocyte count. In the viral infection, the immune system of the body cannot eradicate the virus. The latter actually becomes a part of the lymphocytes. The individual with the infection may be an asymptomatic carrier. Evidence at this time, although still incomplete, would indicate that about 25-30% of these carriers develop ARC, AIDS Related Complex.

In the latter phase, those who develop the complex may suffer from headaches, fatigue, fever, enlarged lymph glands, dry, persistent cough, diarrhea, and weight loss. These symptoms may persist intermittently for years. Those with widespread enlargement of lymph nodes are said to have PGL, persistent generalized lymphadenopathy. In this phase, depending again, on many health factors, the viruses are destroying more of the defensive large lymphocytes the T4 Cells, CD4+, (Helper T1/2-cells). Some researchers believe that changes in the body may accelerate this destruction due to an autoimmune reaction, an allergic response to infected Helper T-cells. This triggers loss of other elements of the body's immune system, the person becomes very susceptible to what are termed "opportunistic infections", and/or unusual cancers. It is as a result of secondary infections that most patients with AIDS usually succumb.

In homosexuals, 60% of whom have protozoan parasitic diseases, it commonly is from one of these that fatality occurs. The terminal infections may be common bacterial, viral, or fungus infections. Tuberculosis, coliform, streptococcal, staphylococcal infections, influenza, herpes, hepatitis B, and crytococcosis are the more common ones. Ordinarily these infections are relatively mild or benign but in AIDS, with the loss of the body's defense system, they overwhelm and destroy the individual. One of the most common infections is due to the protozoan, pneumocystis carini. In a person with a normal immune system it might cause a mild pneumonia from which the patient usually recovers promptly. In AIDS patients, the outcome is quite different. In PCP, pneumocystis carini pneumonia, the organisms grow in the respiratory tract and meeting with no resistance, they multiply rapidly, spread and overwhelm many patients.

Sulphonamides and other drugs are now being used to treat these patients with some success. Unfortunately, there are many recurrences. AZT, Zidovudine, is now being used in an effort to prevent them.

Another invader, toxoplasma gondii, likewise a protozoan parasite, is commonly found in AIDS patients. It usually invades the brain resulting in dementia and eventual death. The cytomegalus virus, CMV, can also be deadly. Infection with the cryptoccocus, common in the environment, often results in meningitis.

A somewhat different type of disease found, particularly in homo- and bi-sexual men with AIDS, is Karposis sarcoma. Ordinarily this is a benign, mild form of cancer characterized by small dark blue or purplish brown plaques initially on the feet and ankles. In AIDS patients, these plaques spread rapidly, involving the hands and arms. The cancer spreads through the lymphatic system. It may cause bleeding in the intestinal tract. It, too, is generally fatal in AIDS patients. The HIV prepares the soil for the devastating secondary invaders.

The symptoms of AIDS patients then, are similar to those of the ARC, AIDS related complex stage, but are more severe and are complicated by additional symptoms caused by the opportunistic infections. Persistent infections of the mouth, oral thrush, dementia, memory loss, and depression often occur. Positive blood tests confirm the diagnosis.

Will all persons infected with HIV develop AIDS? Unless effective treatments are found that will destroy the HIV, it is now thought that most individuals harboring the virus will develop AIDS within five to ten years. Lifestyles will influence this. Time alone, will provide us the final answer.

What treatments are available for HIV infected persons? Currently there is no known cure, no drug, or other means of destroying the virus once it has gained access to, and infected, the body.

The FDA has approved use of the drug AZT, zidovudine, marketed as Retrovir, as being effective in prolonging the life of AIDS patients. It is likewise being used in individuals infected with HIV, but who have not yet developed symptoms of ARC or AIDS, to delay the onset of symptoms. The drug is expensive, costing about six thousand four hundred dollars per year, per patient. Smaller doses of the drug, 50% of that now being used, may prove to be equally effective. Unfortunately, 50% of AIDS patients cannot take AZT, Retrovir, because of side effects. Use of Probenecid, a drug effective in treatment of gout, or alpha infection, in conjunction with AZT is thought to enhance the effectiveness of AZT and further reduce the cost of treatment. Other drugs, DDI, didianosine, and ddc, Zalcitabine have been approved for use with AZT.

Recognizing that an estimated million or more persons in the United States are harboring the virus, with forty to fifty percent of these on the verge of developing symptoms and with forty to fifty thousand suffering from AIDS, the costs of treating all of these are staggering.

Another approach in treatment has been transplant of bone marrow. Thus far, this has only been successful in identical twins. In addition to drugs, research is being carried on to find a vaccine to prevent infection with HIV. Dr. Jonas Salk is now testing a "killed vaccine" on volunteers. Variations in the form of the virus pose a major problem in this effort. Supportive treatment, adhering to good health practices, avoiding possible infections, and combating opportunistic infections in patients who have progressed to the AIDS stage, are essential to treatment. Many hospitals, health departments, and AIDS treatment centers provide diagnostic treatment and conduct clinical studies and research. The Federal government is providing hundreds of millions of dollars to finance such projects.

Prevention is the most important measure we have to combat HIV.

As I have said, for those who have acquired the infection, the course of the disease will be influenced to a great extent by one's lifestyle. Limiting sexual contact to one partner, safe sex, using condoms, avoiding the use of alcohol, tobacco, and abusive drugs, maintaining a well-balanced and adequate diet, enjoying enough rest, and 7-8 hours of sleep a night, minimizing stress, and getting a moderate amount of regular exercise, are all important in either avoiding or in combating HIV. Those harboring the infection should not ingest raw milk or foods that might possibly be contaminated. They should avoid questionable water supplies and persons having contagious infections. It is important to maintain good dental health and personal hygiene. One should see his own physician or visit a clinic every six months. Taking AZT and other drugs would depend on blood test findings.

Understanding and support of the person having a positive blood test for HIV infection is very important. Obviously the afflicted individual suffers from considerable stress, is worried about the future, and needs support and reassurance.

What is the risk to those who are not infected and how can they avoid getting the disease? To answer this question we must look at the reservoir of infection and recognize that different segments of the population are at greater or lesser risk. The majority of infected persons are found in homo- and bi-sexual males, 70-75% of total cases, and in intravenous drug abusers, 20-25% of reported cases. Haitians are now considered to be a high risk group. Babies of infected mothers suffer major potential to become infected. About two hundred and fifty children have been found to have AIDS. Seventy-five percent of these received infections from their mothers. Studies thus far show that approximately 50% of homo- and bi-sexual men have a positive blood test for antibodies to the virus. the incidence in IV drug abusers is even higher.

As mentioned earlier, the greatest concentration of reported cases initially was found in the San Francisco and New York areas. Los Angeles soon joined there ranks and now reports of cases of AIDS are coming from the majority of the states. Most of the cases in the United States occur in men, over 90%. It is interesting to note that one third of the female sex contacts of infected males have antibodies to the HIV. One half of female IV drug abusers test positive for the antibodies. Prostitutes as such, are not necessarily infected, but many of them do use drugs and some have been exposed to infected bi-sexual men.

Again, blood from persons infected with the virus and semen from infected males are the vehicles for the transmission of the infection. Male homo- and bi-sexuals practicing anal or oral copulation are particularly vulnerable. Common use of hypodermic needles and syringes among drug abusers, and sharing of earrings among them are dangerous practices. Crude, rough tattooing using pins and pens can spread the virus in high risk groups. Promiscuity increases the hazard of acquiring the infection.

A great deal of fear has been engendered about AIDS patients and persons known to be infected with the virus. Fear is justified in high risk groups. For the rest of the population, in heterosexuals there should be concern in the promiscuous and awareness of the disease by everyone. More heterosexuals are becoming infected. Actually the hazard of the HIV carrier to the general public, including casual contacts in the home, is very slight. There have been two reports of professionals infecting their patients. One report involved a dentist, and another a surgeon. These reported instances are being thoroughly investigated by the C.D.C. Likewise, there have been isolated cases reported in health personnel as a result of accidental needle sticks, about one in every two hundred such incidents. Although the virus occasionally has been found in the saliva and tears of persons harboring the disease, no one has ever been known to have been infected through contact with them. As stated earlier, the HIV must be encased in a blood cell for transmission. Alone it cannot multiply and it loses its ability to infect. The hazard of receiving contaminated blood or blood products as mentioned earlier, largely has been eliminated with the chance of contracting the infection through them being less than one in a million. Theoretically, mosquitos, fleas, and other bloodsucking insects could transmit the infection, but it is very unlikely. No such transmissions have ever been reported.

Precautions that might be taken in a home where one of the members is known to be infected are largely, those of good hygiene. Use of individual towels and toothbrushes and sanitizing dishes, glasses, and tableware is sound practice but probably has little to do with spread of the virus. The latter is readily destroyed by 25% alcohol, ordinary chlorine bleach solution and by common commercial disinfectants. A sex partner of an infected male member of the family should be particularly careful to avoid semen of the male. Proper use of condoms is protective, though not a one hundred percent guarantee against infection.

A question often arises about marriage when one of the couple has a confirmed positive test for HIV infection. That is most difficult to answer. Marriage would be possible but a prospective bride or groom should be fully informed about the infection and the hazard to one's mate. He or she should know of the possibility of the partner developing AIDS or ARC and of the sorrow that would result. Other problems relating to having a child should be fully discussed. A woman or a man willing to assume the risks involved might be found but such a person would be an unusual one. State, or other law might prohibit such a marriage until a measure is found that would prevent transmission of the infection.

The government is greatly involved in combating AIDS. In addition to financing detailed clinical studies, research for a successful treatment, and some preventive measure such as a vaccine, it is conducting widespread education programs about AIDS and how to prevent acquiring HIV infection. More programs are being planned. Clinic services and hospitalization are being provided. Screening and blood testing for antibodies to the virus are being offered to high risk groups and persons having symptoms suggestive of infection with the virus. This supplements screening of potential blood donors and others.

When one considers the cost of hospitalization of one AIDS patient for 3-6 months during his or her terminal illness, amounting to $50,000.00 to $100,000.00, and then projects this cost based on the expected number of AIDS patients requiring hospitalization in just five years, the total would exceed several billion dollars in one year alone. This would not include clinic, laboratory, and other related medical costs. Nor would it include the incalculable costs in terms of pain, suffering, sorrow, and death; and the loss of productivity of those afflicted and of their families. Total costs can be staggering.

The obvious answer to minimize this problem is PREVENTION. We should be doing a great deal more of it nationwide, for both economic and humanitarian reasons. We should learn of symptomless carriers through greatly expanded blood testing programs. We should learn of, and check on, their contacts, and advise these contacts on measures they can take to prevent the spread of infection. Cooperation of carriers and contacts cannot be obtained alone by laws, regulations, or public education. It must be obtained on an individual basis by skilled health personnel. Some counseling and contact tracing is being provided, but far too little. David E. Rogers, MD., Vice-Chairman of the National Commission on AIDs summerized the current situation accurately, when he stated, "In attempting to control AIDS, we have failed to develop any national prevention program worthy of the name!"

What could be done to establish a good preventive program? We have excellent models of programs used in the control of syphilis and tuberculosis. Fifty years ago syphilis was widespread. The best estimates concluded that a minimum of one percent of the population was infected with the disease in one of its many forms. Tuberculosis was likewise rampant. Fifty percent of all adults had positive skin tests, showing prior infection with the tubercle bacillus, (not active tuberculosis). Health departments played a major role in controlling these diseases.

Unfortunately, today, we have too few local health departments. Only a small portion of the total population has the benefit of their services. If we had adequately staffed Health Departments, massive programs of early diagnosis; treatment of cases; counselling of cases and contacts; and epidemiologic investigations could be carried on. Such a program would supplement the essential role of the private physicians.

By establishing the confidence of patients, staff learn of contacts, find them and arrange for testing and treatment as indicated. The skilled public health nurses, aids, and special investigators, as well as public health physicians, supplementing counseling of their patients by private physicians, are able to explain effectively the manner in which these diseases are spread. The record of control, of tuberculosis, syphilis, and other infectious diseases attest to the success of such control programs. Obviously, effective means of treating persons with infections once located; cooperation; diagnosis and treatment by private physicians; and the educational programs of the National and local Tuberculosis Associations as well as the American Social Hygiene Association; were major contributing factors in attacking syphilis, and tuberculosis.

Similar approaches could be made in attacking AIDS, and in preventing the spread of HIV. They are being carried on in some centers and in some communities but unfortunately, many health departments have been so fragmented and staffs so decimated that they cannot provide the necessary service to duplicate the successes achieved in controlling other communicable diseases. Many areas of the country have never benefited from the services of an adequately staffed local health department.

This deficiency in well-organized, completely integrated, community based public health services for our entire nation constitutes one of our greatest weaknesses and unfortunately, is hardly recognized as we attack the AIDS pandemic.

Formerly, health departments were entrusted to control communicable diseases such as AIDS. Now control of AIDS, has become a political issue with recommendations of epidemiologists and public health physicians, if sought, often being disregarded. In the meantime, AIDS continues to spread.

5. Role in Control of Tuberculosis*

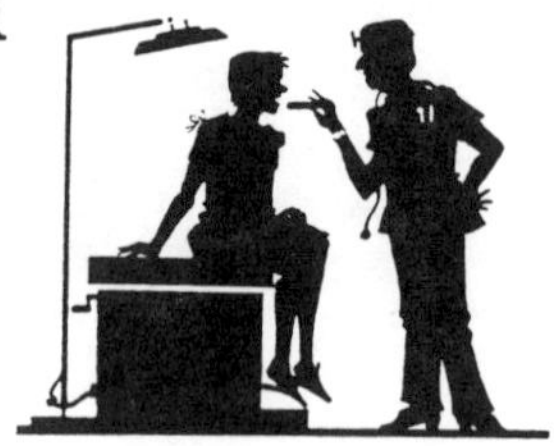

"THE WHITE PLAGUE"

At the beginning of this century this disease was one of the most sinister of communicable diseases, threatening, disabling, and killing millions of people of all ages. It was not spectacular in its destruction but it was an insidious reaper of death. It has been recognized for centuries as "consumption". Galen, a Greek physician, suspected that it was communicable but his suggestion had little impact and was lost until Robert Koch in Germany, in 1882, discovered the tubercle bacillus and proved beyond a doubt that it was the cause of tuberculosis.

As stated, at the beginning of this century, the disease was labeled as the White Plague in Europe. Other appellations by which it was known include apical catarrh, phthisis, consumption, and tuberculosis. The disease had been killing millions throughout the world. It was thought to account for one quarter of all deaths at that time.

During the eighteenth and early nineteenth century, consumption, or phthisis, was accepted as somewhat inevitable and as a pleasant way to die. Treatment of terminal patients with opiates probably added to this belief. The disease was associated with genius since many great artists, musicians, and writers of the time were afflicted with it. Contracting the disease and anticipating an early death, (most died in their twenties or thirties), may have stimulated some to make the most of their lives while they still had a chance. It is true that many dazzled the world with their artistic creations. One writer who supported this belief stated, "The same fire which

*I have gone into more detail explaining the history of the disease and about its control because it **clearly** illustrates the potential of Health Departments in control of communicable disease.

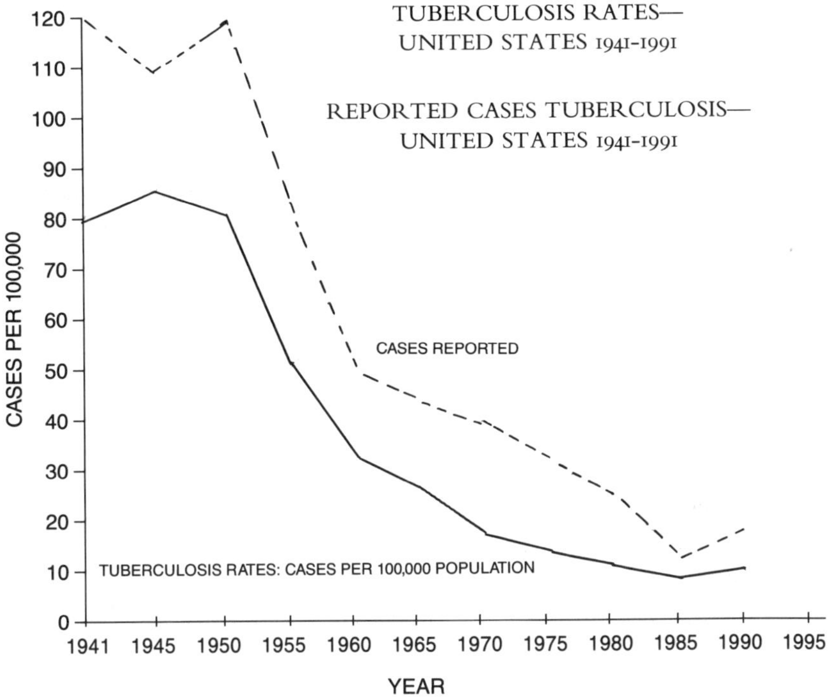

wastes the body in consumption also makes the mind shine with a bright light," Mozart, the famous Austrian composer, died of it at the age of thirty-five. Robert Louis Stevenson, John Addington Symonds, and Elizabeth Barrett Browning, famous writers, also died of consumption. In upper class society consumption was thought to enhance women's beauty. To the poor however, consumption was more realistically thought of as the cause of much poverty and a great killer.

Koch's discovery of the cause of the disease brought about a radical change in attitude toward tuberculosis and toward those who had it. Now it was recognized as a blot on society. Those infected were considered unclean, others thought that these poor victims were being punished for their sins. Great fear of this widespread killer developed primarily because there was no effective medication for it. Comprehensive, accurate data is not available but in New York in 1882, almost one of every thirteen persons was thought to be afflicted with tuberculosis.

The most common form of the disease was the pneumonic type

involving the lungs.* The other forms involved bones, intestinal tract, and lymph glands. These resulted from drinking raw milk from cows infected with bovine tuberculosis. Involvement of the spine often resulted in a severe curvature or hunchback, so well portrayed in the film "Hunchback of Notre Dame". Gradual acceptance of the value of pasteurizing milk, and later (1917-1935), the successful eradication of tuberculosis in cattle virtually eliminated these more unusual forms of tuberculosis in humans.

Some advances in the treatment of the pneumonic form occurred with the establishing of Open Air Sanatoria. the first of these, a colony, was established in the late 1880's at Saranac Lake, New York, by Dr. Edward Trudeau. He had contracted the disease from his brother and, expecting to die, he traveled to Saranac Lake to enjoy the mountains that he loved. Amazingly he began to recover. Soon he was leading a normal life. He became a forceful proponent of fresh air, bed rest, and a good diet including lots of milk, fresh eggs, and red meat.

Those consumptive patients who could afford this care flocked to the sanatorium. Many did recover. The success of this type of treatment was widely recognized as documented in an editorial in the Journal of the American Medical Association, February, 1905.

> Home and Sanitarium Treatment. The open air treatment of tuberculosis is today an established fact. Its curative value is proven beyond cavil. It is not an experiment. It does not mean, however, that the patient is to be restored simply by a few weeks or months sojourn in a lodge in some vast wilderness or out-of-doorlife at a fashionable mountain resort or a tent life in his own back yard under the simple guidance of his own sweet will. It means rather, a systematic, regulated life under rigid discipline and routine. It means constant watchfulness of every symptom . . . (by a well-trained professional staff).

I remember hearing of patients in these open air sanatoria in New York and Colorado who slept on open porches even in the midst of winter with flurries of snow over their beds. Drs. Ralph and Roy Matson, acknowledged chest specialists in the early part of this century operated such a sanatorium

---

*Described as a quick consumption resulting in early death in contrast to the more usual chronic form. Persons having the characteristic cough, night sweats, low grade fever, weight loss, and related symptoms in the later stages of the disease were easily recognized. In early stages some of the affiicted thought they had "bad colds", but the symptoms didn't clear up.

for many years just a few miles from Portland, Oregon. Here the patients enjoyed nature's well-humidified air and rain in the winter months, rather than snow. I'm not sure whether the extreme cold and snow of New York or the milder temperature and rain of Oregon was the more effective. Certainly rest, a good diet, and the relaxed atmosphere in a beautiful wooded area near the Willamette river in Oregon were conducive to improvement.

With this success, state governments were encouraged to establish state tuberculosis hospitals or sanitoria where known infectious cases of tuberculosis could be sent for similar treatment and equally important, to isolate them from other members of their families and the community. This markedly reduced the spread of the disease. Many states did establish such hospitals. Oregon had three of them. The first was established near Salem, the second in The Dalles, and a third, the University Tuberculosis Hospital, in Portland. The latter, built in the forties, was devoted largely to the care of advanced cases requiring surgical procedures.

The State of Washington, with the encouragement and leadership of Dr. Cedric Northrop, Director of Tuberculosis Control, established many county tuberculosis sanitoria of pavilions throughout the state. Excellent care was provided and with the conveniences and proximity of these facilities to the homes of patients, a large portion of those needing such care received it. Care was often free as tuberculosis was a pauperizing disease and most patients could not afford to pay the minimal charges billed by the state.

An equally important development early in the century was the organized effort to inform the public about tuberculosis, how it was spread, and the importance of early diagnosis. The National Tuberculosis Association was established in 1904 and soon Christmas Seals became a familiar reminder to most households throughout the nation of the prevalence of tuberculosis and the need to finance control measures. Health education measures characterized by such slogans, "Taters comes from Taters and Tuberculosis comes from Tuberculosis", and films on tuberculosis, such as "Behind the Shadows", were effective in inpressing people with the idea of infectiousness. Laws to prevent spitting on sidewalks were enacted. Educational campaigns utilizing the press, magazines, speakers, attractive literature, and films were carried on. Some of the messages included were "Cover That Cough", "Destroy Papers Contaminated With Sputum", and of course, "See A Doctor For A Cold That Persists". State and local chapters of the NTA prompted the employment of school nurses, public health nurses, and, starting in the late thirties, the establishment of local health departments. In many instances the Associations helped finance these departments motivating the county governing bodies to establish them.

These nurses and health departments supplemented the public information activities of the Tuberculosis Association by teaching in the schools and providing information to patients referred by private physicians. Public health nurses visiting in homes did a great job in informing families about tuberculosis. In families where a case of tuberculosis had been found, the public health nurses taught measures to prevent the spread of the disease. All of these activities led to better understanding of tuberculosis.

The second major development in control was in improved early case finding and isolation of infectious cases. All over the country, and particularly during the late thirties, with the establishment of many new local health departments, tuberculin testing was done, predominantly in the schools. As health officer in The Dalles, I gave thousands of tuberculin tests.

At that time we found that 5% of the children entering school had a positive tuberculin reaction as did 20% of high school seniors. During the same period, the late thirties, 50% of the adults that we tested in food service personnel examinations and other adult screening programs had positive tuberculin tests.

All of those with positive tests were given full-size chest x-rays. Most of them showed only the primary healed tubercle, but occasionally we found an individual with early or moderately advanced tuberculosis. When a case of tuberculosis was found, or reported by private physicians, family contacts were checked to find the source of the patient's infection, if possible, and to find other members who might also harbor the bacilli. These investigations were fruitful. Follow-up of family contacts of school children with positive tuberculin tests were not productive as the original contact had occurred too long ago to find the source. The trail had grown cold. Infants and pre-school children were checked in well-baby and pre-school clinics. Family contacts of children found with positive tuberculin were examined and often the source of infection was found.

Another case-finding procedure that was helpful at the time was the annual chest x-ray exam. Some states required all teachers to have x-rays and certifications by a physician of absence of tuberculosis. This resulted from the occasional occurrence of tuberculosis in a group of school children where the source of the infection was found to be their teacher. Physicians, nurses, and hospital attendants were known to be at greater risk to infection than others. The majority did have periodic chest x-ray examinations.

In the late forties and early fifties development and use of mini-film, 35mm movie-type film, reduced the cost of chest x-rays and together with widespread campaigns, carried on jointly by tuberculosis associations, medical societies, and health departments, resulted in millions of adults being screened for tuberculosis.

I well remember in the mid-fifties the USPHS had twenty five miniature film mobile x-ray units available to larger cities that wished to conduct widespread tuberculosis case-finding programs. Most of the programs initially, were conducted in the cities on the east coast. Interest grew and larger cities in the central and mid-western areas of the country took advantages of the services.

West coast cities began to participate and some of us in Oregon were interested in having such a program in Portland. Because of the concern of an influential leader in tuberculosis control that such a massive case-finding program would jeopardize the long range local effort, the offer of the USPHS was not accepted. As Oregon State Health Officer, I then explored with the Surgeon General of the USPHS the possibility of including in a survey the residents of the Willamette Valley, an area with many small cities, towns and more densely populated rural areas than in other sections of the state. The Surgeon General and his staff concurred in exploring the feasibility of such a project. It was approved. Because of the outstanding success of this program, due largely to the excellence of the community health education program, mobilization of support of voluntary organizations and the interest of the public I think it is worthy of detailing some of the techniques that were used.

Mary Jo Kraft, a very capable health educator with the USPHS, visited us and organized the program. Her skills in community organization were great. On her first visit to my office miss Kraft—we soon called her Mary Jo—outlined the availability of mobile x-ray units, staff to operate them, read film, and to offer consultation. In addition the USPHS provided supplies, including x-ray film. Mary Jo explained that the chief local contribution would be in arranging for persons to come in for the screening, maintaining records, and doing necessary follow-up. She said that local participants must contribute ten cents per capita for every person screened. This would be equivalent to about one dollar today, considering inflation. I explained that we did not have a budget for the monies and I did not see any way of raising the money until the next session of the legislature. Mary Jo said not to worry about the money, she was sure that it would be raised. She stressed that the important decision was on the need for such a program. I assured her that the need was extant. We than called in key members of my staff including our Directors of Tuberculosis Control, Public Health Nursing, Laboratories, Health education, and Local Health Services. This staff concurred in the necessity for such a program, but they were concerned about finding the matching funds. Again, Miss Kraft assured us that the funding problem would be resolved if the program was needed.

The next step was to consult with the health officers of the eight counties involved. They likewise supported the need for the program, but could not help but express concern as to how the necessary local funds would be raised. Mary Jo again gave reassurance on that score and suggested a series of local meetings in each county involving the local health officers, key members of their staffs, the county court (a three member elected court that administered county government), and representatives of the local medical society, tuberculosis association, and schools. These were arranged. At these meetings enthusiasm for the screening program was tremendous and various bodies offered not only their full support, but also funds for the program! Mary Jo was right. With the assistance of these groups, community organizations were established.

Meetings were held at which the need for and the purpose of the program were explained. Plans for use of the mobile x-ray units were developed. Within a short period of time every known organization in the area was involved, including medical, dental, and nursing associations; Kiwanis, Lions, Rotary, Exchange and other service clubs; PTA's, League of Women Voters, Federated Women's Clubs; Boy Scouts, Girl Scouts, YMCA, Grange, schools, social workers, churches, Chambers of Commerce, and Unions. Enthusiasm continued to grow. It was amazing how communities responded with determination to make this effort an outstanding success. Promotional materials including well-illustrated and simply stated facts explaining tuberculosis and the value of screening, were distributed.

Literally, every doorbell in the Valley was rung, every door knocked on, and every adult was given the opportunity to have a chest mini-film. As a result of this kind of community involvement and cooperation, 80% of all eligible adults in the entire Valley were screened. In some counties percentages rose to 85% and 90%. When one considers that only half of the eligible voters turn out for presidential elections and only 80% of the public registered for sugar rationing during World War II, this was a phenomenal success.

County health officers in Oregon were so impressed with the community organization techniques of Mary Jo Kraft that many of them requested funds for a health educator on their staffs in their next budgets. County courts concurred.

The use of mini-film in this type of mobile unit program, as well as in stationary clinics, advanced screening and also aided greatly in follow-up. Efforts were always made to determine if suspects had active disease.*

Prior to the use of mini-flim in Wasco County, Oregon, where I was the Director of the Health Department, it was a major task and an expensive one to have full-sized chest x-rays taken of both the five percent of school children found with positive tuberculin tests and screened adults. The Health Department had to be resourceful.

We were fortunate in Wasco County in having the Eastern Oregon State Tuberculosis Hospital located in the area. Through the cooperation of its director, Dr. James Odell, and his staff, children and adults who otherwise would not have had chest x-rays, received them. About 15% of the children with positive reactions were found to have active infections. Only 3% required care in a "Preventorium", a nursing home type of facility for children with early tuberculosis. The rest were followed by our public health nurses and generally were x-rayed annually until their infections were healed. Households with children having active primary infections were checked for tuberculosis. An effort was made to follow not only those discharged from the tuberculosis hospitals, but also persons who would not accept hospitalization.

On occasion this was difficult. I remember one family that kept moving. We kept relocating and isolating the family because the father had a positive sputum, was infectious, and he would not permit his rather sickly-appearing pre-school children to be checked. After several moves during the course of many months, the family left our county. We reported this to the state health department expecting that the family would be found

*It was known that many persons, usually in childhood, after intimate exposure to an individual with infectious tuberculosis developed a primary tubercle, ordinarily in the upper part or apex of the lung. Fortunately, most children, and some adults, developed sufficient immunity to encapsulate and surround the small focus of infection with scar tissue and wall it off with calcium deposits. In some cases the individual's resistance to do this was not sufficiently great to isolate the infection and the disease spread. In either event the individual usually became tuberculin positive.

before the father exposed others, and his children became seriously ill. In a somewhat similar case, we finally convinced the parents to permit us to examine their six children. Four of them were of school age. Two of the children were found with early active tuberculosis and were sent to the Preventorium. With good care they recovered. Another instance where the individual failed to cooperate occurred in the early fifties. I was serving as Oregon State Health Officer. One of our local health officers called me to obtain assistance in isolating an older patient who had active tuberculosis with positive sputums. She was a Christian Scientist and although she submitted sputums for examination she insisted on going shopping and visiting neighbors. Her home had been quarantined. Rather than involve the police, I called the state representative of the Christian Scientist church and explained the problem. He assured me that although "his people" did not believe in disease they did believe in complying with the law. He said he would visit the lady and try to obtain her cooperation. He made a 500-mile trip to see her and apparently his presentation was more effective than ours, since the patient ceased shopping personally and did her visiting by telephone.

One of the perplexing problems was that of persons with positive tuberculin skin test reactions who would not accept a chest x-ray. It was available to them without charge if they did not prefer to see their own physicians. On interviewing some of these myself and after explaining the importance of the x-ray, a few occasionally would respond with the comment, "If I have tuberculosis, I don't want to know about it". One wonders why they had the tuberculin test?

One of the really tragic types of cases was the occurrence of miliary (like millet seeds) tuberculosis and of tuberculous meningitis. These, although rare, usually, occurred in infants and young children. Occasionally an adult with an overwhelming infection developed miliary tuberculosis with minute lesions throughout the body, including the lungs. The cases of tuberculous meningitis in infants were sobering. I remember seeing a few of them admitted to the hospital, usually in a coma. There was little one could do for them as we had no effective treatment at that time.

As a result of this screening and follow-up, many previously unknown cases of tuberculosis were found and brought under treatment and observation. Contacts were checked. As a result of these control programs tuberculosis which had been one of the ten leading causes of death, not only in Oregon, but through out the United States, declined dramatically.

Positive tuberculin tests in high school seniors dropped from 20% in 1938 to less than 1% in 1980.

It soon became evident that x-ray screening of the total population was not finding enough new cases of tuberculosis to warrant the effort and cost. Attention was directed to special risk groups, those persons in institutions, prisons, and jails, and to what were called "skid row" residents. The incidence of tuberculosis was still significantly high in these populations to warrant case finding. Many times it was difficult to motivate the alcoholics and other residents of poor hotels and apartments in dilapidated areas of the cities and towns, and the homeless to accept a chest x-ray. In Portland, Oregon, the Multnomah County Tuberculosis Association came up with the novel idea of offering free beer to all who came in for a chest mini-film. The response was tremendous. New cases of tuberculosis were being found. Unfortunately for our case finding, the Oregon State Liquor Commission learned of the program and ruled that such a practice was illegal. No more free beer.

Now that the majority of cases of active tuberculosis had been found, the need for more effective treatment was even more urgent.

In the mid-thirties there were some advances in treatment of pulmonary tuberculosis. Individuals with serious involvement of one lung were treated by collapsing that lung to prevent spread to the other.*

In the early fifties, streptomycin was tried. It was some-what effective but occasionally there were severe reactions to it. Isoniazid (INH) was introduced in 1952. It was quite effective but when used alone, bacterial resistance developed. P-Amino salicylic (PAS) was then tried. Alone it was not particularly effective but when used with Isoniazid (INH) the combination proved to be the most effective yet found.

With time superior drugs were developed and today Ethambutol and more recently, Rifampin, a semi-synthetic antibiotic, have largely replaced PAS for use with INH. Patients with active disease and positive sputums usually became non-infectious within two months of starting to take the drugs. Most returned to their usual activities after the two months.

The majority of patients who have had tuberculosis must be followed

*This was done by repeated injection of air between the rib cage and the affected lung or by temporarily paralyzing the phrenic nerve by a "phrenic crush", If these measures failed, a thoracoplasty was performed, removing portions of ribs on the involved side to permit the chest wall to collapse on that side. The latter was a radical measure but it often stopped the spread of infection and did save lives.

with periodic chest x-rays for at least five years. After that with any recurrence of symptoms relating to the lungs, the individual is again checked. Many of these patients are treated on an out-patient basis in clinics and require no hospitalization whatsoever. In addition, within a relatively short time, positive sputum patients become non-infectious and their health permitting, they are allowed to return to their usual activities.

Actually, a significant reservoir of tuberculosis that we have in the United States today, aside from the major one of refugees and immigrants, is that of persons who had a primary tubercle in earlier life. When such a person experiences a serious illness, and a drop in resistance, there is a possibility of the tubercle organisms being freed, multiplying, and spreading. It is important that physicians, health departments and the general public be aware of this hazard.

In many other countries where tuberculosis is much more prevalent, the disease is often occurring in a drug resistant form. Thorough physical and x-ray examinations of these new residents should be made and treatment and appropriate control measures instituted.

As a result of the success of research, diagnosis, treatment, and control programs, savings in lives, and dollars have been tremendous. Problems still remain, however. The fire was under control, but we are now experiencing flare ups.

In the entire United States in 1976, only 2,419 deaths occurred from pulmonary tuberculosis and there were only 711 deaths from other forms of the disease. In 1979, tuberculosis cases numbered 27,817 for the entire United States as reported to the CDC. You may well remember that in the beginning of this century, it was estimated that twenty-five percent of all deaths were due to tuberculosis. If the same rate applied today, we would have about 325,000 deaths in one year from all forms of tuberculosis. The actual number was 3,130 which is less than 1% of the expected number if the initial rate had prevailed.

Case finding and treatment (particularly of refugees), good housing to prevent overcrowding, and good nutrition are important to prevent spread. We do not have as effective a vaccine to prevent tuberculosis as we had for smallpox. Physicians and health departments must be alert and active in control.

6. Attacking Other Threats to Public Health

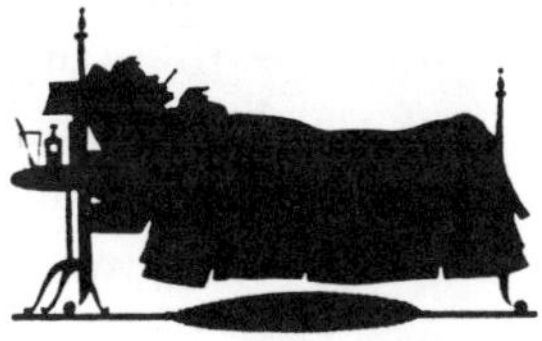

THE ZOONOSES
ANIMAL DISEASES TRANSMISSIBLE TO MAN

ANOTHER TYPE OF disease with which physicians, veterinarians, and health departments have been particularly concerned are the diseases of animals transmissible to man.

RABIES*

Rabies, or hydrophobia, an infection resulting from the bite of an infected animal, is the most serious of the Zoonoses. Rabid skunks and bats are the most hazardous to man. Dogs, wolves, and foxes may be infected, and rarely cats, cows, and horses. Prior to 1885 rabies was universally fatal. Imagine the alarm after a dog bite. Would the person bitten suffer a horrible death from hydrophobia? If stricken, there was no treatment for it. In July of 1885, Louis Pasteur vaccinated a boy who had been bitten by a mad dog, against rabies. The boy survived. Shortly afterward, a French bacteriologist, Pierre Roux, demonstrated rabies virus in the blood. Spread to the brain and nervous system accounted for the symptoms. Prevention and control of the disease became possibilities.

Depending on the location of the bite, number of bites, and severity, the incubation period of the disease can vary from one to several months.

*Symptoms beginning with local numbness at the site of the bite is rapidly followed by a severe headache, irritability, difficulty in swallowing and breathing, and great thirst. Strangely, there is fear at the sight of water, which is how the earlier designation, hydrophobia, came into common usage. Anxiety and restlessness increase. These symptoms are followed rapidly by muscle spasms, convulsions, delirium, and coma. Death often occurs within two to three days.

Prevention has been effective through education of the general public as to the hazards of rabies, vaccination of dogs against the disease, prompt reporting of bites by dogs, skunks, or bats, and administration of anti-rabies serum or vaccine shortly after the bite, if laboratory examination of the brain confirms that the animal was rabid. Too often in the past, an uniformed person would kill the suspected animal by shooting it in the head. This usually damaged the brain so severely that an adequate laboratory examination for rabies could not be made. Thanks to education, this does not occur as frequently now. Improved vaccines using duck embryos in the production stages are effective, but there is a slight hazard connected with these vaccines. Even better vaccines are now available. The health officer, the family's physician, and the family often face the difficult decision as to the risk involved in taking the vaccine, weighed against the risk of getting rabies.*

With dog bites, the problem is more difficult. If the dog is known, it is quarantined for at least ten days to determine whether it remains well. If it becomes ill with possible early signs of rabies, the animal is sacrificed without damaging the head. The head is iced and sent for laboratory analysis of the brain. With fluorescent antibody technique, on finding the typical Negri bodies (microscopic bodies in the nerve cells) in the brain, diagnosis of rabies is confirmed and vaccination of the victim of the bite is recommended. Vaccination is usually accepted. The real problem arises when the bite is slight and the dog cannot be found. I remember one such case in Riverside, California. Since the wound of the small child was slight, and since the physician had thoroughly cleansed the laceration and had given a booster inoculation for tetanus and because no case of rabies had been know to have occurred in dogs in the area for the previous twenty years, we concluded that the risk from the vaccine and the cost and inconvenience outweighed the possibility of the boy becoming infected with rabies. The family agreed. The lad was not vaccinated, his laceration healed quickly, and he remained well.

Similar questions arose in regard to bites of bats. Generally the involved bat died, was found, and could be examined. Often in southern California if it is determined that such a bat is infected with rabies, vaccination is recommended. Continued alertness, awareness of the hazard, maintenance of surveillance in wild animals, and vaccination of dogs should keep rabies under control.

---

*In western states skunks occasionally bite persons. As the wild animals cannot be found, and because of known infections in skunks, vaccination is recommended.

UNDULANT FEVER* BRUCELLOSIS

Unfortunately in the past, but rarely now, cows, goats, and pigs can be the source of brucellosis infection in man. Before the need for pasteurization of milk was accepted and before brucellosis was largely eliminated from dairy herds, it was found quite commonly. Three types of brucellosis occurred in animals. Cows were infected with B. abortus (an infection which frequently caused cows to lose their calves). Goats were infected with B. melitensis which cause a more serious illness in humans than that caused by B. abortus. Hogs became infected with another type, B. suis, which was transmitted primarily to farmers or hog producers.

Brucellosis generally tended to be chronic. Occasionally a person with the disease would have an episode of acute illness with fever, headache, and chills. Usually, the symptoms were vague, with general fatigue, loss of appetite, and a low grade fever. The latter might be low during the day, high in the evening, or it could occur for a few days, disappear and then return again, [giving an]undulating type of fever. This pattern accounted for the terminology, undulant fever.

In the late thirties, herds of dairy cows were sometimes found to be infected. I remember a herd near The Dalles, Oregon, that was the source of raw milk for one of the large dairies in the community. Originally, the herd consisted of about one hundred and twenty-five cows. B. abortus infection was found in the herd and eventually the entire herd had to be sacrificed. The federal government helped to indemnify the dairyman. Some infections of humans had occurred because the milk was not pasteurized. Today, there would have been lawsuits. Then, there were none. After this incident, most people in the area demanded and obtained pasteurized milk.

In the late forties, a physician in Portland, Oregon, became very much interested in brucellosis. Other physicians referred patients having suggestive symptoms to this physician for investigation. He reported over fifty cases in one year. Although the Oregon State Health Department did not

---

*The illness was characterized by vague abdominal complaints, joint pains and loss of weight. Some patients had symptoms so vague that they were considered to be psychoneurotics. Diagnosis was difficult in chronic stages as the culture of bacteria from the blood, urine, or spinal fluid was most likely only during the initial stage of infection. Rising titers of agglutination tests (reflecting an increase in the body's immunity to the infection) helped the diagnosis. Until antibiotics became available, treatment was was difficult and primarily supportive. Later tetracycline and streptomycin were found to be quite effective.

request "compulsory" pasteurization of all milk sold in the state, the legislature considered such a measure on the basis of the reported cases. When opponents learned that most of the cases had been reported by one physician, they labeled it a "one man epidemic" and were successful in defeating the bill. Another small outbreak of B. melitensis infection occurred as a result of eating imported goat milk cheese produced from raw milk. Investigation of this cheese and the finding of B. abortus in cheese made from raw milk in the states, led to laws requiring all cheese to either be aged for ninety days or more, or to be produced from pasteurized milk. The aging process destroyed the brucella organisms. Pasteurization was equally effective. As a result of these measures, the testing programs, and elimination of infected animals, brucellosis is now quite rare.

PSITTACOSIS-ORNITHOSIS
PARROT FEVER

Another Zoonoses, acquired from birds, is psittacosis in humans, (ornithosis in birds). Psittacosis was the name given to a viral disease which had been known to occur primarily in persons working in aviaries, usually with imported parrots. Occasionally it caused a serious pneumonia-like illness often resulting in death.

In the early part of the century there was no specific treatment for the disease. Regulations were adopted limiting the importation of parrots. In the early thirties it was recognized that parakeets could also be a source of the infection. These little "love birds" were very popular with their gay colors and ability to learn to repeat a few words. Thousands were imported into the United States from Mexico and Central American countries. States adopted regulations strictly limiting import to legitimate, long-time pets and to birds from aviaries maintaining high standards of cleanliness and surveillance. Because of the profit potential (parakeets could be purchased for as little as fifty cents apiece in Mexico and then sold for twenty dollars or more in the states), smuggling of illegal parakeets became fairly common.

One episode that I recall involved the smuggling of several hundred parakeets packed in egg cartons and in egg cases. A truckload was brought into southern Oregon. The dealer buying the birds lost many of them due to ornithosis, and she herself became ill. The discovery of this incident gave the state health department an opportunity to locate the smuggler, seize a truckload of infected parakeets and thus stop the distribution of these diseased birds.

Another outbreak of psittacosis was discovered in Portland, Oregon, in the early fifties as a result of the alertness of a young physician at the Veterans Hospital in Portland. One of the doctor's patients had a rather severe type of pneumonia. He was given the usual therapy with antibiotics, fluids, and bed rest, but he did not respond to the treatment. Tests for many related kinds of illnesses were made but these all proved to be negative. The doctor persisted in his efforts to diagnose the illness and reviewed the history of the patient. He learned that the man worked in a turkey processing plant near Portland. Knowing that infection with the psittacosis virus could occur in turkeys, and that the infection could be transmitted to man, the physician asked the Oregon State Health Department to investigate the turkey plant. Monroe Holmes, D.V.M., our veterinarian, checked immediately and found that many of the turkeys being processed showed evidence of ornithosis. About thirty persons in the plant had recently been ill with "severe colds" and pneumonia. Six of them had been hospitalized. Some of the office staff had been infected as well as the workers in the plant. Investigation revealed that particles of the high pressure water spray used in the process of dressing the birds, had been carried through the air conditioning system to the offices.

Two ranches and several thousand turkeys were involved. The turkeys were a special breed, broad-breasted bronze. Those being processed were confiscated. All turkeys on the two ranches were killed and buried. Some two thousand turkeys already processed, packed, frozen, and readied for shipment to military camps were quarantined for several months until repeated checks showed them to be safe for use if properly cooked. No infections resulted from their release and use.

Fortunately, treatment with tetracycline and chloramphenicol resulted in prompt recovery of both the patient at the Veterans Hospital and the others involved. The diagnosis of psittacosis had been confirmed. This serious outbreak of psittacosis and ornithosis would have been completely overlooked had it not been for the persistence and astuteness of the doctor at the Veterans Hospital who brought about the inquiry at the turkey processing plant and the epidemiologic efforts of the state board of health.

Limitation of the import of rare birds, reasonable assurance of freedom from ornithosis of those imported, and continued alertness of physicians, veterinarians, and the general public to the disease have resulted in an almost complete eradication of these infections in the states.

TRICHINOSIS*

There is another group of Zoonoses, the Cestode or worm infections. Included are tapeworms, roundworms, whipworms, and infection with their larvae. We will only consider trichinosis. A dramatic occurrence of acute illness in the families or groups eating improperly cooked trichina-infested pork was not uncommon in the late eighteenth and early nineteen hundreds. Homemade sausage utilizing pork as the main ingredient, was a particularly hazardous food when curing was substituted for adequate cooking. Undoubtedly many isolated cases of trichinosis occurred in the population and were not diagnosed because their symptoms were minimal, due to having ingested only small amounts of the trichinous pork. Autopsy studies in the twenties revealed that probably twenty to twenty-five percent of the total population experienced infection with trichina.

The encysted or encased larvae of a minute roundworm, trichinella spiralis, are spread through the meat, or musculature, of the pigs that become infected predominantly from eating scraps of meat from other trichinous animals. It was found that bears as well as hogs also could be infested. Thorough cooking of the meat, or freezing at sub-zero temperatures for a period of days, destroys the larvae.

Illness in the more severe cases results from the dissemination of the trichina larvae in the musculature of the body. In severe cases death frequently has occurred. Treatment is largely supportive.

A classical case recently was reported when a well-known actor, Yul Brynner, who allegedly became infected after eating what was thought to be insufficiently cooked spare ribs at a well-known restaurant. In this instance a lawsuit followed, charging negligence of the restaurant for inadequately cooking the pork. According to the press, a sizeable settlement was made.

Major control of the infection has resulted from two major public health

---

*Presence of the larva in the intestinal tract, in the eye muscles, diaphragm, shoulder, and other muscles of the body result in pain and difficulty in contracture. Nausea, vomiting, cramping, and diarrhea usually occur within two to three days. Depending on the number of larvae ingested, chills and fever follow later with difficulty in swallowing, speaking, and vision. Symptoms due to involvement of the brain, heart, lungs, and nerves may last for a period as long as a month.

measures. The first involves public education. Most people, including restaurant operators and cooks, are aware of the hazard of eating improperly cooked pork and assure that it is cooked adequately. The second is the control and limitation of the practice of feeding uncooked garbage to hogs. For many years, in an attempt to reduce the incidence of trichinosis, health officers recommended to legislatures that they adopt laws to prohibit the feeding of garbage to hogs (particularly in commercial operations) unless the garbage had been heated to a temperature sufficient to destroy trichinae. Probably because of opposition by hog ranchers who fed garbage to hogs, legislatures failed to enact this legislation until outbreaks of "virus exanthem" began occurring in hogs in the late fifties. Investigation revealed that the disease of hogs was spread through the feeding of uncooked garbage. Thousands of hogs died of the disease. When this information was made known, and because of the threatened economic loss, farm interests now requested legislatures to enact laws requiring the cooking of garbage fed to hogs. Within two years most states that had rejected the proposal on the basis of protecting humans from trichinosis now enacted this type of legislation.

Fortunately, humans also benefited from the requirements to protect hogs and today trichinosis is rather rare. Where were our priorities? Protecting hogs appears to have been more important than protecting humans!

Recent occurrences have been traced to eating home-smoked sausage. The importance of adequately cooking pork cannot be over-emphasized.

INTESTINAL INFECTIONS
SALMONELLOSIS*
PARATYPHOID FEVER

Initially, Salmonellosis was thought to be a mild form of typhoid fever but it is now recognized as a separate entity caused by Salmonella. There are some nine hundred serotypes of Salmonella, the most common being S. typhimurium.

Salmonellosis was not one of the plagues feared so much at the beginning of this century, in fact, it was not recognized as an entity. Although these infections are less serious than typhoid they still cause rather severe

*Symptoms vary from mild to moderately severe. They consist of fever, abdominal pain, nausea, vomiting, and diarrhea lasting for three to five days. The disease usually is self-limited. Antibiotics are reserved for the more seriously ill.

illness and occasionally death, particularly in debilitated persons or in small children. They are often called food poisonings although, strictly speaking, they are infections. Contaminated water, raw milk, and occasionally cracked eggs, meats, and other foods contaminated by carriers or rodents, eaten raw, or inadequately cooked have been the source of infection.

We won't go into detail on symptoms but it is worthy to note that while the incubation period of typhoid fever is from one to two weeks, the onset of symptoms in Salmonellosis is usually from twelve to forty-eight hours. The organisms must multiply in the body. Occurrences often involve only a small number of persons, but larger outbreaks have occurred predominantly as a result of contaminated water supplies. An outbreak in which I was involved in during the early forties occurred at a Kaiser shipyard in Portland, Oregon. The water systems on newly built ships were tested by flushing them with Bull run water, Portland's very pure municipal supply. A huge valve controlled a connection between the public water supply and Willamette River water. The latter supply was to be used only in case of fire. The river serves as a large inland port for many ocean going vessels. It was known to be contaminated. Unfortunately, during a fire drill on the ship, someone turned the huge control valve permitting polluted Willamette river water to be drawn into the potable water system. This contaminated most of the supply line for the shipyard. As a result, over 2,000 shipyard workers became ill with the salmonella infection.

Another outbreak, probably the largest Salmonella outbreak that has ever been reported in the United States, occurred in the early sixties in Riverside, California. I was then with the California State Health Department. We were called in to assist in the investigation, along with epidemiologists and sanitary engineers from CDC.

The water supply came from deep wells. the water was of excellent quality. As chlorination of deep well water was thought to be unnecessary, the supply was not chlorinated. The possibility of contamination in the distribution system had not been fully appreciated. Almost 20,000 people residing in Riverside became ill within a matter of days. At first the local health department staff believed the outbreak was some kind of food poisoning, but as the number of of reported cases increased and the distribution was studied it was realized that only the public water supply could account for the widespread occurrence and the number of cases. Directions were given to the public to boil all water before using it for drinking purposes. Very few secondary cases were reported.

Most of those who became ill experienced typical symptoms of Salmonellosis. A number of individuals, particularly infants and the elderly, required hospitalization, and a few deaths were attributed to the outbreak. Although epidemiologists, sanitary engineers, sanitarians, and other staff members of the CDC, state and local health departments, studied the outbreak for several months, attempting to determine how the contamination occurred; the source of the contamination was never discovered. It was suspected that the water supply could have been contaminated by a break in the water mains under chicken ranches, or cross-connections in industry. Even sabotage was considered. but none of these possibilities could be shown to be the cause.

The best possible explanation was demonstrated later by Laura Elliot, Director of the Laboratory of Riverside County Health Department. She had learned that redwood chips in water, would sustain growth of Salmonella in the laboratory. She was aware of the existence of a large reservoir in the Riverside water system that had been out of use for several days and that had been put back in service a few days before the outbreak. She discovered that there were some redwood floats in this reservoir. Was it possible that the reservoir could have been the source of the infection? In 1970 the city planned to discontinue use of the reservoir. Laura conferred with the director of the water system on the possibility of testing out her theory. He agreed. As Riverside County Health Officer, I approved of the experiment, provided that all connections of the reservoir with the public water system be severed and that the reservoir not be used again. These provisions were accepted. The reservoir was filled. A rather minute quantity of Salmonella culture, about the quantity that could have been introduced by a mouse or bird, was placed in the water. Daily checks were then made of water samples from the reservoir to learn whether Salmonella could be recovered. The organism was recovered after the fourth and through the tenth days. To remove any doubt, after a period or several months the experiment was repeated. Again, after inoculating the water in the reservoir with a minute amount of Salmonella, positive cultures for the bacteria in increasing numbers were obtained on several successive days. It seemed that this reservoir, with its redwood floats, the contents of which had not been used for several days and which had then been put back into service could have been accidentally inoculated from natural sources. As the water was not chlorinated and with the nutrients provided by the redwood, the organisms could have grown and been distributed inadvertently through the public water system when the reservoir was put back into use. Although it was recognized that the cost of installing chlorination equipment in such deep well water supplies was great, state department of health policy was changed to require such chlorination. Riverside, California, as well as other communities in the state with deep well water supplies now chlorinate them.

Another major outbreak of Salmonella poisoning occurred in early 1985 in mid-western states. It was centered around Chicago, Illinois. Over 11,000 cases were reported including several deaths. The unusual aspect of this was the fact that it resulted from a breakdown in the pasteurization process of raw milk. A large dairy in suburban Chicago was implicated. Several employees in the dairy were found infected with Salmonella. A large food chain retailed the milk.

The Illinois Department of Public Health was criticized for delays in initiating steps to control the outbreak. It is significant to note that neither the Illinois State Health Director, Thompson Kirkpatrick, who was discharged by Governor James Thompson, nor the successor, Jerome Margolis, appointed by the Governor, had a background in health. Later, as a result of public pressure, the Governor appointed Bernard Turnock, M.D., a qualified public health physician, as Director.

Occurrences of Salmonellosis were traced to raw milk distributed by a large dairy in southern California. The health department, based on the results of epidemiologic investigation, stopped distribution of the raw milk until the source of the contamination could be proven. Subsequently the dairy prevailed on the state legislature to enact a law that prohibited the health department from taking such action unless the Salmonella organisms were actually found in raw milk specimens. The health department has been able to do this in recent occurrences and has taken necessary action prohibiting sale of the contaminated, unpasteurized milk until the source of contamination could be found. This is an illustration of how health departments can be handicapped in protecting the public health.

SHIGELLOSIS*

Another waterborne, milk or food borne infection is shigellosis. It, too, can be serious.

---

*An intestinal infection rather similar to Salmonellosis.

An occurrence of Shigellosis took place in the Palm Springs area of California in the early seventies. It illustrated not only an outbreak of shigellosis but in addition, how deceptive the appearance of water can be as to the presence of bacteria.

Several cases of Shigella dysentery were reported from the area. The health department laboratory confirmed the presence of Shigella in the stools of young people who were afflicted. They were obtaining water for drinking and other purposes from a crystal clear little river which cascades down from the mountains towering above Palm Springs. The river flowed through a recreation area which at that time did not have a water supply or restroom facilities. Some young people had climbed the steep canyon along the river to camp, many for several days.

Our sanitarians took samples of the water. We expected to find E. coli bacteria which would show pollution from human or animal excreta. To our amazement we not only found E coli, but we also found Shigella organisms. Rarely are the disease causing organisms found in a natural state of this kind. As we could not control the use of the river for drinking, we closed the area for recreational use. No further cases of Shigella dysentery occurred in that area.

GIARDIASIS

During the early part of this century the presence of Giardia lamblia, a type of protozoa, was not considered to be particularly serious as the organisms were often found in the stools of persons who apparently had no symptoms of the disease. In recent years occurrence of rather severe intestinal illness has been attributed to Giardia.

One such outbreak was reported in the early seventies in Colorado. Since then, many cases have been reported in other states. A typical case occured in 1972, in Riverside County, California. A physician from a small resort area called me to ask my advice on the diagnosis and treatment of one of his patients suffering from severe diarrhea, alternating with constipation, generalized weakness, and loss of considerable weight. The patient had been ill for several weeks and had been hospitalized twice. The usual tests and examinations for intestinal infection had been negative. Antibiotics were of no value. I suggested that blood and stool examinations be repeated. Again they were negative.

About two weeks later the doctor called again in desperation, seeking assistance in the diagnosis as the patient was still very ill, losing more weight, and was not responding to any treatment. In the meantime I had read of the unusual outbreak of giardiasis in Colorado. Symptoms were similar. I suggested that stool specimens be sent to our health department laboratory. We checked and found the cysts of Giardia. With this information, the doctor began treatment with atabrine. The patient immediately began to improve and completely recovered.

This may have been an unusual case but it illustrates the need to consider such an infection when the more common causes of an intestinal illness are not found. The health department laboratory played an essential role in the case.

AMOEBIC DYSENTERY*

Another intestinal infection not commonly seen in the United States but still prevalent in many developing countries is amoebic dysentery. The protozoan organism, Entamoeba histolytica, responsible for the disease, can result in mild, almost imperceptible symptoms, or in severe illness often resulting in death. It is contracted from drinking polluted water, ingesting contaminated food, or from a carrier. The latter emit cystic forms of the amoeba in their stools and thus transmit the infection.

In the forties and fifties, a number of cases were encountered in the United States. Many of these were thought to be the result of eating contaminated lettuce imported from Mexico.

Travelers in developing Asiatic, Central and South American, and African countries need to be aware of the hazard of this and other infectious disease. They should protect themselves from the dysenteries by eating only thoroughly cooked foods, or fruits that can be washed with treated water and personally peeled. They should use only actually boiled or otherwise treated water for drinking or brushing teeth and they should not neglect thorough cleansing of the hands before eating. Ice, ice cream, and dairy products should be avoided in developing countries.

I am sure that many of us have personally experienced such infections, or have friends whose trips in developing countries were ruined by

---

*One of the more serious types often involves the formation of abscesses in the liver. Due to the color of the contents, these were called chocolate cysts. Unless treated, and even with treatment, this form can be fatal. The dysentary type of illness can vary from mild to severe forms in which ulceration of the intestinal tract frequently occurs.

acquiring this or other types of intestinal infection. A physician friend or mine and his wife took a tour of southeast Asia in the sixties. They enjoyed themselves but the wife, upon her return, had bouts of intestinal upset, eventually proven to be amoebic dysentery in a chronic form. Although she had the best possible treatment available she developed cysts of the liver and months later died of the disease.

Now treatment is quite effective but different drugs must be used for different forms of infection. Again, prevention is the best precaution. After spending two years in India without experiencing any of the intestinal infections I can assure you that they can be avoided, even without offending one's hosts.

CHOLERA*

Cholera, another intestinal infection, is seldom seen in the United States although it, too, still occurs in developing countries where water supplies are often polluted and foods may be contaminated. Caused by bacteria, Vibrio cholerae, the illness can be severe. The mortality rate until the latter part of this century was as high as 75 to 80 percent. Vaccination is somewhat successful. Although its complete effectiveness is questioned, it certainly is advisable to take it if one plans to travel in countries where cholera may occur.

To control the disease, health authorities attempt to vaccinate everyone in the area where cases of cholera are occurring. It was interesting to me to witness a cholera vaccination program in northern India in the late sixties. Thousands of people were making a trek on a narrow road leading to a sacred Hindi shrine. The health authorities had set up a "clinic" in a small pass on the trail. Each traveler reaching the point was asked to bare his or her arm. The "vaccinators" with large syringes of vaccine proceeded to inoculate each one. There was no provision for sterilizing needles or syringes. the prime objective was to vaccinate every passer-by as quickly as possible.

I was thankful to have had my vaccination in the United States. Apparently the operation was successful as the outbreak subsided. With

---

*The typical rice water stools and accompanying dehydration, unless promptly treated, can result in death within a few days.

improved sanitation, vaccination and better treatment this serious infection is being controlled worldwide.*

No deaths from cholera have occurred in the United States since the forties, and the few cases that have were contracted in other countries. Again, awareness of the hazard, and taking precautionary measures, including vaccination, protects against the disease.

HEPATITIS

In discussing infectious intestinal diseases we must include hepatitis. There are two major types, one, an intestinal viral infection involving the liver, and the other an insidious viral infection usually transmitted in blood, most commonly when dirty syringes and needles are shared by drug addicts.**

The first type of hepatitis has been a problem in institutions, particularly for the developmentally retarded. Poor personal hygiene contributes to its spread. Improved sanitation and hygiene have been effective in its control. the second type caused real concern due to its transmission through blood transfusions and because of the hazard to medical personnel. It can be sexually transmitted, as discussed earlier. Through blood testing and development of a Hepatitis B virus vaccine, the hazard from this type of virus is being reduced.***

UNUSUAL INFECTIONS OF PUBLIC HEALTH CONCERN
ROCKY MOUNTAIN SPOTTED FEVER****

Rocky Mountain Spotted Fever was first encountered in the Rockies west of the Cascade Mountains in Oregon and Washington, and the Sierras in California. In this area it was caused by the bite of a rickettsia infected wood tick. In recent years it has been found that a similar infection in the southern part of the United States is transmitted by a dog tick.

Education on avoiding ticks, wearing protective clothing, checking for ticks after exposure, and an effective vaccine have largely limited the

---

*Recent means of combatting dehydration have been very successful.

**AIDS can likewise be transmitted.

***Currently, Hepatitis accounts for more deaths than AIDS. It is estimated that over 300,000 cases are occurring in the United States each year. Up to 10% of these become carriers.

****The symptoms are somewhat similar to those typhoid fever, but with a rather typical generalized rash.

infection. When given early, antibiotics reduce the severity of the illness and chance of death in those who acquire the disease.

LYME DISEASE*

Although this infection also results from the bite of a tick, a very minute one found on deer, other warm-blooded animals and birds, it is not caused by rickettsia, but by a corkscrew-shaped bacteria, a spirochete.

The incubation period of Lyme Disease may be from a few days to years. Treatment with antibiotics should be given promptly. If not diagnosed early**, neurological invasion can result in death. Several thousand cases have been reported from most parts of the country in the past few years. Precautionary measures to prevent infection are similar to those for Rocky Mountain spotted fever. A vaccine to protect against the disease is now being developed.

Q FEVER

Q Fever is a relatively rare disease caused by another rickettsial organism. It is acquired through breathing dust contaminated with the organism, or, rarely, from ingesting infected milk. Cattle, goats, and sheep are often infected (as are humans) in dry arid areas where dust from cattle and sheep ranches can be carried into the air. The symptoms can be similar to those of flu. In this case antibiotics are not as effective as in many other infections. They can only supplement the value of rest and good diet.

Valley Fever (Coccidiomycosis), likewise rare, is also contracted through inhaling contaminated dust.

Although not ricketsial, coccidiomycosis, and histoplasmosis, both caused by fungi, are diseases that can be confused with flu. They may be mild or quite severe. An antibiotic such as Amphotericin B, has been found to be useful in their treatment.

Informing the public of the hazards, and recommending pasteurization of milk (Q Fever) have been the public health measures used to combat these diseases.

---

*Usually the first symptom is a rash followed by flu-like symptoms.

**Use of a D.N.A. test of spinal fluid is quite accurate in diagnosis.

LEGIONNAIRE'S DISEASE

This disease is mentioned, not because it is widespread, but only because it was unique epidemiologically. An unusual outbreak of flu-like disease following a large meeting of Legionnaires, baffled physicians and health department staffs for months. It finally was discovered that the infection was spread through the ventilating system of the meeting hall.

These accounts of unusual infectious diseases emphasize the variety of problems that health departments have faced and are facing, in protecting the public's health.

TETANUS AND GAS GANGRENE

Two infections of a different type which resulted from contamination of wounds from soil were feared because contracting one of them meant an almost certain, painful death. These infections are tetanus and gangrene.

Both infections were more common in the United States than bubonic plague. Tetanus, commonly called lockjaw, is now largely controlled through preventive measures and moderately effective therapy if the infection is recognized early. Wounds of a crushing type are most serious. Spores of an anaerobic bacilli, (clostridium tetani), found in the soil, cause the infection. Piercing of the skin with a rusty nail was thought to be particularly hazardous. The bacteria inhabit intestinal tracts of many animals. Soil was contaminated frequently by horses on farms, in rural areas, and in cities where they were used to pull carriages, wagons, and even streetcars.

A classical case of tetanus resulting in death occurred in 1924 when the son of President Calvin Coolidge blistered his heel. The broken blister became infected, young Coolidge developed tetanus and died although he had the benefit of the best medical care available at that time.

Use of tetanus globulin or tetanus antitoxin at the time of injury, if the individual has not been immunized against the tetanus, has further reduced mortality from this disease. With the reduction in the use of horses as draft animals, with knowledge of the source and hazard of infection, and with the use of tetanus toxoid as an immunization agent, incidence has become very low.

Gas Gangrene occurred most commonly amongst the cavalry and other soldiers during early wars when horses were used. With limited use of horses and the introduction of modern antiseptic treatment for wounds, this infection with one of the Clostridium bacteria, has become a rarity. An antitoxin has been developed for use in gas gangrene but it is not very satisfactory. The fatality rate is still high when the infection occurs.

FOOD POISONING
PTOMAINE POISONING

True food poisonings are the result of ingesting food containing toxins or poisons that have developed in the food prior to eating it. This results from contamination with bacteria. In the early part of this century sudden illness after eating contaminated food was called ptomaine poisoning. Correctly speaking the latter refers to poisoning from alkaloids resulting from the putrefaction of meat or other nitrogenous food. It is rare.

STAPHYLOCOCCIC FOOD POISONING

In the early nineteen hundreds we began to differentiate types of food poisoning and found that staphyloccic food poisoning was the most common one. It is caused by toxins formed in foods that have not been properly refrigerated. Turkey dressing, Hollandaise sauce, certain cream pies, egg and ground meat mixtures and other perishable foods can be contaminated with staphylococci from the nose, throat, or an infected wound, (usually on a finger). At ordinary room temperatures the bacteria grow and within a few hours, produce a toxin which does not change the taste of food. When ingested, severe symptoms can result.

Until the hazard was well-publicized, outbreaks of "staph food poisoning" were quite common. I remember in the early fifties, members of a large union and their families had a picnic on the Sandy River near Portland, Oregon. The food for over one thousand people was catered. Within two to four hours after eating, many became ill with nausea, vomiting, profuse sweating, weakness, cramps, and diarrhea. Inadequate refrigeration had permitted staphylococci, accidentally introduced into the food, to grow. Toxin had been produced with dire results.

Another similar episode occurred in the early fifties in connection with evacuees from the Columbia River, Vanport, Oregon, flood. A small group of people was being housed in a church being used as a temporary shelter. The local chapter of the American Red Cross was providing food. Volunteer workers, not acquainted with the hazard of staphylococcic food poisoning had prepared delicious ground meat and mayonnaise sandwiches for a lunch. A few were leftover and put aside.

As some of the older evacuees had enjoyed the sandwiches so much and as they did not want a big dinner, they were served the sandwiches that had been left from lunch. The sandwiches had not been refrigerated. Within two or three hours these "seniors" became violently ill. As a volunteer physician and Oregon State Health Officer, I was called to see them. Those that were ill were sweating profusely, vomiting, suffering from diarrhea, and weakness. Some were in shock and had blood pressures so low that it was difficult to obtain their pulse. We hospitalized four of them. Fortunately, they all recovered. Subsequently, strict standards were established by the group providing for greater care in the preparation of sandwiches, selection of the types of foods used, and the discarding of any remaining foods that could not be properly refrigerated.

Restaurants, bakeries, and other commercial businesses generally are well aware of the hazard of staphylococcic food poisoning. They take precautions to protect foods as required by health departments. The occasional outbreaks of food poisoning are usually in family or group gatherings where volunteers prepare the food, where the hazard is not recognized, where the refrigeration facilities are inadequate, and where health departments are not responsible for supervision. Health departments seek to prevent such outbreaks through health education and promotion of high standards in commercial food preparation, storage, and serving.

BOTULISM

This is another type of food poisoning largely controlled through protection of food preparation. It can be fatal when it occurs. Again, before the cause was known, in the late eighteen and early nineteen hundreds, isolated cases of death from eating home-canned non-acid vegetables, meat, or fish, occurred in the United States. This type of illness had been described in Germany over one hundred years earlier. In those instances it was related to sausage making. In this country bacteriologists recognized that botulism organisms found in the soil, grew in certain non-acid canned foods when improperly processed. The spores of the organism were not killed by boiling and when the jars were sealed, the vacuum and lack of oxygen resulting, provided an ideal condition for the botulism bacteria to grow and produce

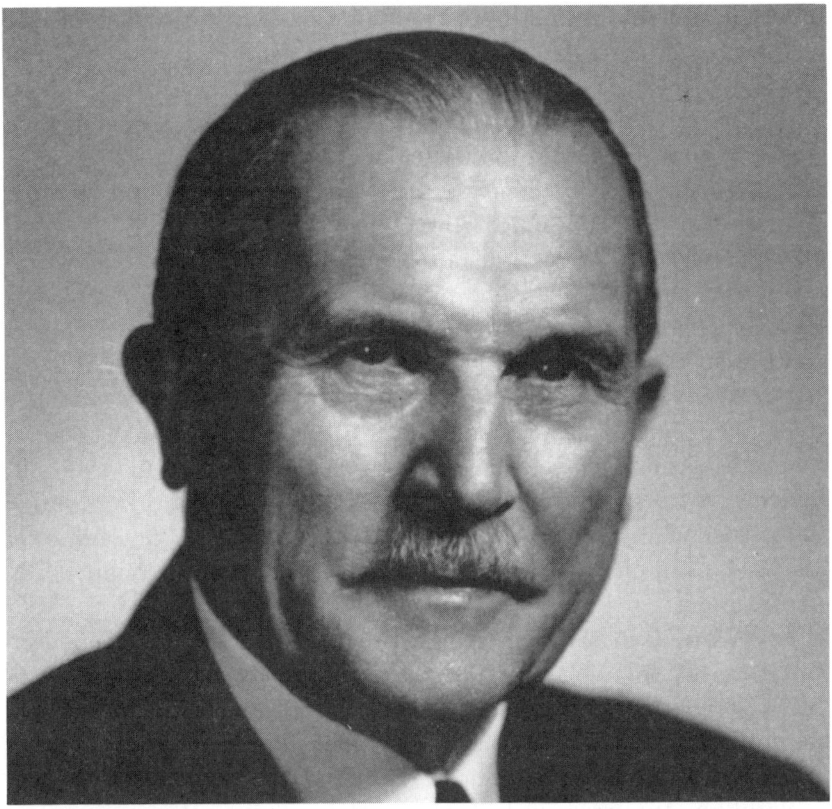

Dr. Karl F. Meyer

toxin. It can be deadly. It has been reported that chefs and other persons have died shortly after merely tasting a contaminated, improperly processed food such as olives or string beans containing botulism toxin.

Some difficulty occurred in commercial canneries in the early part of this century, particularly in the processing of olives. Illness and deaths as a result of eating canned olives threatened the canned olive industry. Dr. Karl F. Meyer, an authority on botulism, was called in. He established standards for the industry, providing for pressure cooking for prescribed periods of time and at given temperatures. Following the adoption of these processes, not only in California but throughout the nation, no further cases of botulism occurred for over forty years.

To Dr. Meyer's dismay, an incident occurred in the 60's to sully this remarkable record. An outbreak of botulism resulting in several illnesses and death, occurred after eating canned tuna fish.

The source of the canned tuna fish was traced to a packer in San Francisco, California. All of the canned tuna from that plant was recalled by the U. S. Food and Drug Administration. Dr. Meyer was called in again as a consultant. A thorough investigation was made. Records showed that all of the cans of tuna fish had been properly processed. Only a few cans of those recalled showed contamination. It was thought that some cans might have been packaged without having gone through the "cookers", but this possibility was ruled out. Although it could never be proven, it was concluded that the most likely cause was the use of a lighter metal can than that used by most processors, incomplete sealing at the joint between the cover and the side seam, and the drawing into the can of botulism spores that somehow had contaminated the cooling water. In any event, under the strictest supervision, about fifty tons of canned tuna were buried deep in one of the San Francisco Bay Area dumps. Further safeguards were established and no further cases have been reported from commercially canned foods.

Physicians and most people are now familiar with the hazards of botulism and with the symptoms which develop shortly after ingesting the toxin. Nausea, vomiting, appearance of double vision, difficulty in speaking and swallowing, followed by difficulty in breathing due to paralysis of nerves governing breathing may occur.

Botulism antitoxin is available and is life-saving if the diagnosis is made early and the antitoxin is given promptly. Health departments generally can make the antitoxin available or have it brought in rapidly by airplane or through the cooperation of state police.

Until means of prevention and treating these food infections and food poisonings were developed, many thousands of persons became ill or died as a result of eating contaminated foods. Now, as a result of establishing standards for food processing and maintaining these standards through public health surveillance, foods are preserved safely. In the rare instance where the safety net fails, prompt action is taken by health departments to remove any questionable food, make an investigation as to the cause of the failure, and institute prompt action to correct the problem. The major hazard now is from foods canned in foreign countries where our health departments cannot control the canning process. The U.S. Department of Agriculture has been unable to examine sufficient samples to eliminate this problem.

Because control of this type of outbreak illustrates so well how the health department team functions in such an emergency, I will briefly describe a typical operation to control one.

The first reports of probable victims on an outbreak received by the clerks are immediately brought to the attention of the health officer and the epidemiologist, if the department has one. After conferring with the reporting physicians and confirming the diagnosis, the department staff is mobilized. With appropriate laboratory tests, and often by visiting afflicted persons, a determination is made as to the kind of an outbreak that is occurring, its extent, and the potential for spread. The public health nursing staff, sanitarians, health educators, and statistical staff are alerted as well as laboratory personnel. Pin maps to show location of cases are often prepared and studied. Representatives of all units of the department meet with the health officer to review the problem and to determine what action each of the staff is to take in gathering additional data, alerting the public and instituting control measures.

Subsequently timely meetings, often daily, are held to review progress until the outbreak is under control. All appropriate staff members functioning as a team contribute to the action. Depending on the type and extent of the outbreak, officials of the government, other department directors, state health department, and CDC are informed. Every resource of the department, and others as indicated, is mobilized. This type of team action has been the basis for success in attacking such public health problems in the past.

In effectively limiting all of these diseases the importance, in fact, the necessity of having an adequate team of specially trained and experienced health department staff is obvious.

7. Contributions in Control of Nutritional Deficiency Diseases

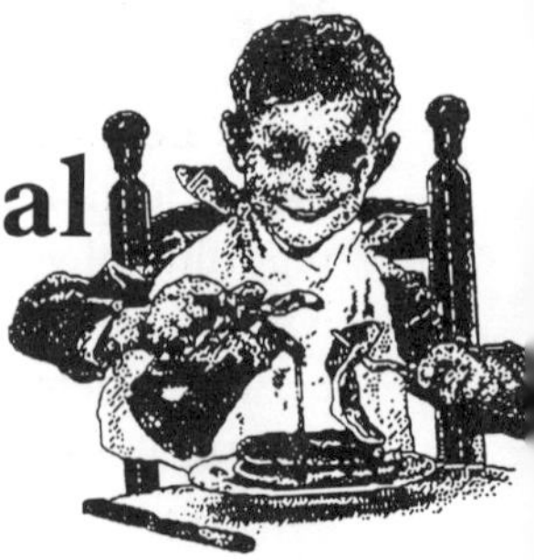

ANOTHER GROUP OF diseases that health departments have been very much involved in their control are the nutritional deficiency diseases. First, let us look at scurvy.

Although James Lind, in 1735, had discovered that feeding citrus fruits would cure scurvy, it was not until 1885 that the existence of scurvy was proven. Later, Lind's findings were confirmed and through widely publicizing this and through health education in the schools, the disease was largely eliminated.

In the early 1900's, a disease was observed in the south-eastern portion of the United States similar to that previously found in Europe. It was serious, resulting in death of about two-thirds of those afflicted. It was called pellagra.* Concern increased. In 1909, a Nutritional Conference on pellagra was convened. The consensus was that it was infectious. Surveys showed it to be more common in children, women and the poor.

In 1914, Dr. Joseph Goldberger, a USPHS officer, was called to Mississippi to help control an outbreak of pellagra. He was told by other physicians that it was an infectious disease. He doubted this. During his investigation, Dr. Goldberger observed that only the younger boys in an orphanage developed the disease. Older boys on a work force seemed to be immune. Why? Dr. Goldberger checked on various aspects and learned that the diet of the two groups differed. Because they worked, and it was thought that they needed it for energy, the older boys were given meat, milk, and eggs in their diets. The younger boys, because of cost, were fed primarily carbohydrates, potatoes, rice, and grits. In 1915, Dr. Goldberger suggested

*Symptoms included a skin eruption, initially like a severe sunburn, intestinal upsets, dizziness, and in severe cases, dementia.

that all children in the orphanage be given diets including meat, milk, and eggs. No further pellagra occurred in the orphanage.

Dr. Goldberger then obtained permission from the Governor of Mississippi to recruit volunteers from the prison to determine if pellagra could be produced by diet. He assured the Governor that no drugs would be given. The prisoners were aware of the hazards of the disease, including the possibility of death. Eleven convicts volunteered. They were fed the usual diet of many poor people in the south, at that time, potatoes, rice, and grits. After six months, six of the prisoners had developed early pellagra. There were still dis-believers. To prove beyond a doubt that the disease was not infectious, Dr. Goldberger, a co-worker Dr. Wheeler, and Mrs. Goldberger were given blood from a woman with advanced pellagra. None of them developed the disease. The dietary basis of the disease was thus established. But how could poor people afford the improved diet? Studies of dogs showed that adding brewer's yeast to their diets would prevent Black Tongue, a disease in dogs similar to pellagra. Trials of adding brewers yeast to diets of patients in state institutions showed that this addition would prevent the disease. This was a practical solution. Unfortunately, Dr. Goldberger died in 1929, before his studies could be completed. Studies were continued and in 1937, nicotinic acid, the pellagra preventor, PP vitamin, was found by Elvehjem and associates.

Beriberi, another dietary deficiency disease, was found more commonly in the Orient where polished rice was a mainstay of the diet. It did occur in a milder form in this country. Dr. Charles Hose, in 1890, was the first to conclude that this was a nutritional disease. Cusimir Funk showed that rice polishings would prevent it. He extracted Vitamin B1, thiamine, from the polishings of rice, and named the first vitamin. The disease* occurred in this country under conditions similar to those causing pellagra.

Vitamin B2, riboflavin, the lack of which causes a form of dermatitis, body weakness, and eye problems, is a condition again occurring when diets are deficient in protein-rich foods, and particularly milk. Toward the end of this century, these conditions were seen chiefly in alcoholics, whose diets generally are deficient in essential nutrients. It is also found in some of the developing countries.

One of the pioneers in nutrition, Dr. Elmer V. McCollum, was one

*Loss of appetite, muscle cramps, with heart involvement, swelling of tissues, and paralysis occur in advanced stages.

of the first to use animals in dietary studies. He worked with rats and in 1912, discovered Vitamin A, the lack of which results in night blindness. Later, he discovered Vitamin D deficiency, which is one of the factors in the cause of rickets. Dr. McCollum emphasized the value of good nutrition with a well-balanced diet.

In addition to vitamin deficiency diseases, there are other deficiencies in the diet that can cause illness or disability. One of the common ailments in the early part of this century was having a "goitre," an enlargement of the thyroid gland. This condition was found to be the result of an insufficient amount of iodide in the diet. When the problem was publicized and the advisability of use of iodized salt was made known through health education, this malady largely disappeared. The need for other minerals in the diet, including calcium, potassium, iron, zinc, copper, and magnesium is well-recognized now. Today we know of more than thirty vitamins in addition to a number of minerals, essential to good health.

Public health researchers and epidemiologists discovered dietary deficiencies and their relationship to disease. Utilization of this knowledge required a great deal of health education to impart the information to the public and to assist the public in changing their dietary practices accordingly. The combined efforts of physicians, health departments, schools, nurses, dentists, other health professionals, and the media have been quite effective. One of the most productive efforts has been that of the public health nurse or aide consulting with an expectant mother, one having a child, and others in clinics or in the person's own home. This person-to-person consultation on nutritional needs often convinced individuals when other approaches failed.

8. Better Health for Mothers, Infants, and Children

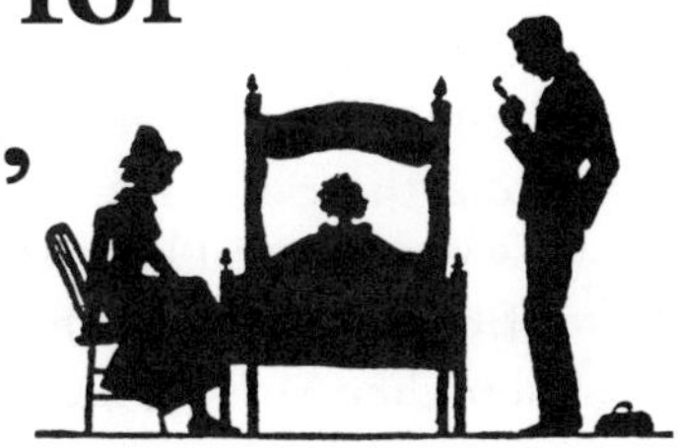

CONTROL OF INFECTIOUS and nutritional disease have saved millions of lives but many other services have improved the health, particularly of mothers, their babies, and children. Many problems have not been fully resolved, especially in prevention. The major deficiency is lack of dollars to support good health department and other preventive health services. It would seem reasonable and an economic measure to divert some of the billions of dollars now spent on medical and hospital care of terminal patients and pre-maturely born infants to preventive health measures.

To fully appreciate some of the progress that has been made in maternal care, we might look at a scene that occurred in the early part of our century as narrated to me by a one hundred year old neighbor. Then I will review some of the developments in maternal-child-health care since.

> "Henry! Henry! Put the teakettle and pan of water on to boil. Put more wood in the stove, then hurry down and tell Maggie Smith to come up as fast as she can. I think the baby is coming!"
>
> Jane watched Henry rush to get things done and then run down the wooden sidewalk to the Smiths. He told Maggie what was happening. She said she would be up soon. She had been mid-wife many times before. Henry made sure the water was boiling. He got out pans, old sheets that had been washed and ironed for the occasion, string that had been boiled, a little blanket, freshly made soap, and a pitcher. He put them on the dresser in the bedroom where Jane was having labor pains. Maggie had arrived. She talked with Jane, reassuring her. Henry paced the floor in the kitchen. He made certain that the kerosene lamps were filled, ready to light. He fixed a bite to eat and made coffee for the three of them. After several hours

> of interminable waiting in silence broken only by occasional cries from his wife, Henry heard the faint cry of a baby. Maggie tied and cut the cord, cleaned up the baby, and spanked its bottom to make it cry again. She called out to Henry, "It's a boy!" After showing the baby to its mother, she handed it to Henry to place in the little crib which he had fashioned from a wooden box.

This was a typical kind of birth in the early part of our century. Very few of these births were recorded except in a family Bible. Aside from neighbors like Maggie, there were few mid-wives trained or experienced in helping mothers give birth to their babies.

I appreciated the incident more when I recalled that a physician friend of mine and I were called to a home in Portland, Oregon in the forties to deliver a baby under similar circumstances. We improvised and successfully delivered the baby, although we were public health physicians, not obstetricians.

Returning to beginning of the century maternity care, in larger cities, women were occasionally admitted to hospitals for delivery. Most mothers however, feared going to a hospital because of the high mortality rates in them. Doctors did go to homes, taking their little black bag and obstetrical kits with them. There were relatively few doctors and travel by horse and buggy was slow. Except in some of the larger cities, few doctors had offices. It was difficult to reach doctors in an emergency since they generally were out making calls. Some interesting stories are told about home deliveries.

In one instance, a doctor was called to a home in the early evening to deliver a baby. He knew the Brown family quite well. At the end of an all night vigil, a healthy boy was delivered. After caring for the mother and the baby, the doctor re-packed his bag, picked up items for his obstetrical pack, gave instructions to the father and mother, and was about to leave when the mother said, "Doctor! Don't leave. I'm sure there is going to be another one." Although the doctor was certain that there was not a twin, he did check Mrs. Brown. He found that she was having contractions again. Hurriedly, he prepared for another delivery and as Mrs. Brown had predicted, in a few minutes he delivered a twin baby girl. After taking care of the mother and baby, and before packing up again, he turned to the mother and said, "And now Mrs. Brown, will there be a third?" This time, Mrs. Brown agreed that it was safe for him to leave.

Not all mothers, or babies were as fortunate in delivery as these. About one mother out of every hundred died at childbirth and only eight or nine of ten babies lived to be one year of age. Hemorrhage and infection were the major causes of death. Sterile rubber gloves were not used until after 1890 when Dr. W. G. Halstad introduced them. Pre-natal care was practically unknown. In complicated cases, without the assistance of a doctor, women occasionally would be in labor for days. It was difficult to believe, but I was told of one instance in the thirties, in which a young mother had been in labor for three days. The family had tried many ways to precipitate the coming of the baby without results. In desperation, one of the family repeatedly jumped on the mother's abdomen expecting thus to push the baby out. Failing in this, the family finally made the twenty-mile trip to fetch a doctor. As one would expect, the baby was dead when the doctor was finally able to deliver it. Actually, the doctor was fortunate to have saved the young mother's life.

As state and city health departments were established, and reporting of births and infant and maternal deaths became more dependable, doctors and women's organizations expressed increasing concern about the emerging data revealing the appalling record of deaths. Sporadic efforts were made to train mid-wives and a few states began to license them. There were a few obstetrical nurses, Margaret Sanger, who was to start the first birth control clinic in 1916, was one of the best known of these.

In larger cities, hospitals began to develop maternity services and a few separate maternity hospitals and homes, the latter usually converted large, old residences. Deaths continued. It was not uncommon to have an outbreak of several maternal deaths from infection. Premature babies had little chance of survival. One can appreciate people's concern. Progress was being made in control of epidemics but obstetrical deaths, a major cause of death nationally, had received relatively little attention. "Occasional" deaths of mothers and babies were accepted as a way of life. Although difficulties in communication and travel made national organization effectiveness cumbersome, women's clubs prevailed on the congress to give this serious problem consideration. In April of 1912, congress established the Children's Bureau. It was given the responsibility of studying the causes of maternal and infant deaths and establishing standards for care and programs to prevent unnecessary deaths.

With the establishment of standards for care in the hospital delivery room, hospital deliveries became more common, recognizing that deliveries in rooms used to care for infected surgical patients was hazardous. Recently delivered mothers could be inadvertently infected by personnel caring for them as well as for other hospital patients in maternity wards, maternity units, or even in maternity hospitals. The importance of prenatal care was being recognized and a few women began to visit a physician early in pregnancy, at least before they went into labor. Advice on diet, weight gain, exercise, and rest was given. In the nineteen sixties and seventies, the hazards of the use of drugs, alcohol, and tobacco, particularly during pregnancy, and the danger to a fetus from German measles, and herpes were emphasized. Women were examined to determine the possibility of complications at delivery, due to unusual positions of the baby, abnormal shape or size of the pelvis of the mother, and physical condition of the mother and to recognize elevated blood pressure, anemia, or other physiological abnormality. Most women saw their doctor at least a month or two before an expected delivery and most had their deliveries in a hospital.

The "county poor" frequently were the ones who received very little prenatal care and who were more likely to deliver on an emergency basis in there own homes. In the twenties and early thirties after World War I, most of the larger counties in the country built county hospitals. Those affiliated with medical schools were often quite good. Others built in conjunction with the "county poor farm" were likely to be of a mediocre quality. County physicians, often employed on a part-time basis, could give only superficial and emergency care. The Great Depression following the stock market crash of 1929, further increased the problem of welfare patients. Economic improvements beginning about 1935, voluntary improvement of hospital care to meet recognized standards, and better education of physicians, nurses, and equally important, of women themselves, were instrumental in reducing both maternal and infant mortality.

The introduction of sulphanilamide and penicillin in the thirties and early forties had a tremendous impact on the treatment of infection. Deaths of mothers due to childbirth infections dropped dramatically.

As we have said, in 1936, congress enacted the Social Security Act and made funds available for the establishment of local health departments. It also made available funds to support special programs in health departments for mothers and children. There were two types of Maternal and child health funds. One for general support, to employ public health nurses, physicians, and to enrich programs for mothers and children. The other was available for special projects, to demonstrate the value of more ideal types of service for mothers and children(such as the Wasco-Sherman County project which I will discuss). As health departments were established, public health nurses were invited to visit homes. They found expectant mothers and encouraged them to see their own physicians early, not in the last trimester of pregnancy, but preferably soon after the individual first recognized that she was pregnant. These nurses did an excellent job. The information which they gave the mothers in their own homes was well accepted and effective. They were able to explain in more detail the instructions of the woman's own physician.

I was fortunate to serve as the Director of a small Health Department in Oregon encompassing two rural counties, Wasco, and Sherman. The population of the two counties at that time, 1938, was only 15,000. We applied to the state for funds for a maternal and Child Health Demonstration. We were given monies to match the funds of the counties and schools to make possible the employment of five public health nurses, one for every three thousand residents, a full-time sanitarian, and a clerk. I served full-time, not as a county physician, but as Health Officer and physician providing only "well-person", or preventive health services. We did not take care of sick people. This surprised many residents but we explained that our job was to prevent illness; to keep people well. However, we did treat individuals having STD. Through education, cooperation with the physicians, schools, voluntary organzations, and the community itself, we actually knew of every expectant mother, newborn infant, and every child in the two counties. To illustrate how comprehensive the program was, one of our public health nurses visiting one of the rural areas, stopped at a service station to buy gasoline. The operator, after providing the gas, asked the nurse if she had seen Mrs. Smith about ten miles distant from this little community. He said, "She is going to have a baby and needs a visit." The nurse did go to see Mrs. Smith, and emphasized to her the need for early pre-natal care. Then she convinced her to see her own physician, and initiated a series of visits to consult with this expectant mother. Later, in cooperation with the woman's physician, the public health nurse helped plan for the delivery.

The physicians as a whole were very cooperative and appreciative of the service; however, I learned that you could not please them all. We worked through the medical society which represented the majority. One of the older doctors with whom I became very well aqcuainted told me of his initial reluctance to refer mothers to the health department for follow-up. He was an excellent physician and did a lot of obstetrics. He told me of a patient who lived on a wheat ranch about forty-five miles from his office. The delivery was complicated and the mother had a tendency to bleed. She was kept in the hospital for about a week to make certain that she did not hemorrhage. Upon releasing her from the hospital, he told her to stay in the city for at least another week and to report back to him immediately if she had any bleeding or other complications. The mother stayed in town for two days at which time she felt so well that she decided to go back to her family and ranch home. She did not tell the doctor of her decision. Two days after she arrived home, she began to hemorrhage severely and before she could be transported to the hospital she died. The doctor was very much upset. He realized then, that if he had informed the health department of the women's condition, a public health nurse probably could have convinced the mother of the necessity of remaining in town, and if not, she would have reported the mother's move to the ranch home and the doctor could have intervened. It was likely that the woman's life could have been saved. The doctor told me that after that experience he referred all of his patients to the health department for public health nursing service. Unfortunately, most health departments did not, and presently do not have sufficient staff to visit all expectant mothers who need such visits.

This type of service and cooperation with the physicians and community resulted in remarkable decreases in maternal and infant mortality rates in those counties and in other parts of the country.

As mentioned earlier, in December of 1941, with the onset of World War II it was necessary to divert physicians, nurses, and other health department staff to military and defense support. Civilian preventive health services were radically curtailed. The congress established the Emergency Maternity and Infant Care Program, the EMIC. Scarce health department personnel were used to administer this major program to assure pre-natal and delivery care for pregnant women, and care for the infants and small children. While the health department did not provide the care, it established standards, and worked out fee schedules with the state medical society. It reviewed reports of care, as well as physician and hospital claims prior to payment. Mothers and babies, all of whom were members of families of men in the military service, received excellent care. Very few complaints were heard from either physicians, hospitals, or patients. It was an outstanding program.

With the end of World War II, the construction of new hospitals began all over the country, stimulated, as we will explain in the chapter on Facilities, by enactment of the Hill Burton Hospital and Facilities Construction Act. Early in this construction program we recognized that many existing hospitals did not meet current standards. Architects found that designing a hospital was quite different from planning an office building, industrial plant, or home. With experience, and with health department advice and supervision, facilities for maternity and infant care were greatly improved to meet acceptable standards.

Great changes occurred in the procedures in hospitals, not only in the delivery rooms and nurseries, but in the practices of serving food, handling of linens, waste, and in staffing patterns. One of the major sources of the spread of infection, particularly in smaller hospitals, was the practice of having one night nurse care for all types of patients in the hospital, including maternity patients and newborn infants. We inspected one small hospital where two mothers had died from infection. We concluded that the night nurse could well have been responsible for spreading infection. Isolation technique often was not used. Another source of spread of infection was the practice of using meal trays, sugar bowls, salt and pepper containers, indiscriminately in various parts of the hospital. The same trays, without an interim washing, might be served to infected surgical, medical, orthopedic, or other patients at one meal, and used for maternity patients at another. Inspections also revealed a practice, in multi-storied hospitals, of placing dirty trays, dishes, and silver in a shelved elevator or lift, removing them, and then without cleansing the shelves, using the same lifts for transporting the next meal to the various floors of the hospital. On explaining the hazards, these practices were changed. Trays were individualized and sterilized after every use and lifts were thoroughly cleaned. Individual salt, pepper,and sugar packets were provided. Similar improvements were made in other techniques.

Plumbing was one of the features health departments checked. The value of these inspections was well illustrated in one incident when the Chief of our plumbing unit in our department in Oregon, Mr. Arthur Farrell, found that a vacuum breaker had not been installed on a new sterilizer in a hospital. After thorough sterilization of packs and equipment, utilizing steam under pressure, the sterilizer was cooled. In cooling, a vacuum developed inside the sterilizer without the vacuum breaker, sewer vapor was sucked back through the drain, contaminating the sterile supplies. This accounted for some of the unexplained infections occurring in that hospital. A vacuum breaker was immediately installed. Previously unexplained infections ceased.

Such things as fire safety and accident prevention requiring safety features like shatterproof glass in nursery windows were not overlooked. Isolation of mothers who had delivered en-route to the hospital, prohibiting visits of small children, improved delivery room techniques; all added to the better care of obstetrical patients and babies.

Many state health departments offered consultation to maternity units from especially trained nurses, expert in maternity and infant care. Hospitals welcomed this assistance. It was one of the most popular services that state health departments offered.

With the advent of penicillin and other antibiotics, mortality from puerperal infections, infections of mothers acquired during childbirth, was again dramatically reduced.

As success of antibiotics in treating infection was recognized, less emphasis was given, unfortunately, to aseptic technique.

During the latter part of the century, as mentioned earlier, more woman sought early pre-natal care and relatively few deliveries took place outside of the hospitals. A few young couples became interested in natural birth in the home and had their babies without a physician's help. Nurse midwives, especially trained, delivered some babies. The latter usually recognized the expectant mother who might have complications and referred these women to a physician for care and for hospitalization. Many hospitals established birthing centers. Mothers were taught to relax and to assist in delivery. This minimized the need for anaesthetics and surgical procedures.

Tremendous progress has been made in pre-natal care, in improving hospitals, maternity care, and in care of newborns. The major problems now are in poverty groups. Increases in accurate sex education in the home and in the schools; intelligent use of family planning to better assure wanted babies and motherhood; and adequate public health nursing and counselling in homes would contribute to even better health of all mothers, infants, and children. Unfortunately, there has been far too little of this personalized type of education.

Thus far we have concentrated on maternal health. What progress has been made in the health care of infants and children? Great strides have been made in preventing early death. The physical and mental health of children has been vastly improved. Infants particularly, benefited from control of the majority of communicable diseases, many of which attacked them. Improved environment, and safer milk and water supplies have benefited them. Early in this century a baby weighing less than five pounds or a two or three months prematurely born baby had practically no chance of surviving. Now, some of the babies weighing as little as 16 to 24 ounces, and even less, are being kept alive to develop into normal adults.

What brought about this dramatic change in the opportunity for a newborn infant to live and thrive? As expectant mothers received better care, and deliveries became safer, not only did the mothers benefit, but the infants benefited too, as standards in hospital nurseries were improved. One of the early problems recognized was blindness in children resulting from infection of the eyes with gonococcus, acquired during birth from an infected mother. This major cause of ophthalmia neonatorum was said to account for 50% of blindness in children early in this century. As explained earlier, laws were enacted to require the installation of drops of a weak silver nitrate solution in the eye's immediately after birth, Crede's method. Now, antibiotics are often used. This practice together with the use of sterile materials in cleansing the eyes of a newborn baby, greatly reduced the incidence of infection and resulting blindness.

Another significant development was the recognition of formula and bottle feeding infants, particularly those whose mother's milk was insufficient to properly nourish the baby. Use of evaporated cow's milk and corn syrup formulas for feeding; recognition of the early need for vitamin C, using orange or tomato juice to prevent scurvy; vitamin D using cod liver oil in the early years and later vitamin D drops, to prevent rickets; cooked egg yolks as a source of iron; and use of strained cooked vegetables, fruits, and meat; greatly improved the growth and health of babies. Now, special formulas are available commercially as substitutes for mother's milk.

One of the innovative and useful programs to supply milk for "premies", and babies whose mother's could not breast feed them, was the development of a "human milk dairy." Dr. Herman Bundeson, Health Commission of Chicago, Illinois for many years, established such a program. He was an astute and innovative public health physician.

I was privileged to visit Dr. Bundeson's department in the early forties and to see mothers express milk from their breasts, and for each mother to provide as much as a quart of milk a day for the human milk pool. These women were paid ten cents and ounce for their milk. Cow's milk was ten cents a quart in stores at that time. The milk was then pasteurized, chilled, and delivered fresh to the hospitals of the city to be used, particularly in feeding premature babies. Excess amounts were frozen for future use. The availability of this milk was life-saving for many prematures until effective artificial milk formulas were produced.

The testing of cattle for tuberculosis and brucellosis, the eradication of infected animals, and the pasteurization of milk was instrumental in practically eliminating tuberculosis of the bowel and bone, undulant fever and other infections which attacked and often killed infants.

About this time in the forties, many states enacted laws, as mentioned in the section on STD, providing for premarital examinations. These included a serological test for syphilis. The requirement was instrumental in reducing the occurrence of congenital syphilis in the newborn. Unfortunately, all states did not enact these laws. Not only resident, but also non-resident couples and their children often suffered as the result of undetected syphilis at the time of marriage in these states.

As infant mortality data was studied, more concerns arose over neonatal mortality, deaths occurring during the first month of life. Infant incubators were installed in many hospital nurseries. These were considered, at the time, to be very expensive, but with there use more premature babies were saved. Health departments were encouraged by the Children's Bureau to provide portable, home-made incubators for home use and for transporting infants from homes to hospitals. In the late thirties, in Oregon in the Wasco-Sherman Counties Health Department, we built four of these little white cabinets. We used screened incandescent light bulbs in the cabinet to keep the baby warm. These did not provide oxygen but the units were well-ventilated. The hinged top had a pane of glass for viewing the baby. These home-made incubators with thermometers, proved to be useful and often life-saving.

Commercial incubators were more refined, with controls for oxygen, temperature, and humidity. Many "premie" lives were saved using these devices. Later, it was found that excess oxygen in some instances had resulted in blindness. With this knowledge oxygen levels were better controlled to prevent retrolental fibroplasia, a degeneration in the eye leading to blindness.

The early advent of vaccines and other immunizing agents against smallpox, diphtheria, whooping cough and tetanus, and more recently against polio, measles, German measles, mumps and chickenpox, further reduced infection from these diseases, complications, and deaths.

The introduction and use of sulfanilamide and penicillin, and use of many additional antibiotics drastically reduced the occurrence and complications of ear infections, mastoid infections, (the bony protuberance back of the ear), osteomyelitis, (bone infection), deaths from common forms of meningitis, and other infections.

As a result of better prenatal care, improved obstetrical care, and more Caesarian sections, when difficult deliveries were anticipated, there were fewer premature births, birth injuries, and disorders such as cerebral palsy. Women in labor were now being monitored to determine any fetal stress, problems in the baby resulting from labor. In the sixties and seventies, more attention was given to genetic diseases. Phenylketonurea, sickle cell anemia, and hemophilia received much attention and were tested for widely. Treatment and genetic counseling for these and other genetic diseases proved helpful. Tests early in pregnancy were used to determine conditions such as Down's syndrome. In the early part of the century this was called Mongolian Idiocy. In some instances the latter condition was found early enough in pregnancy to terminate the pregnancy, if the parents concluded this was best. Using "scans" and other diagnostic techniques, congenital defects such as heart abnormality, occasionally were found. In some instances surgical correction could be made in utero, i.e., the unborn baby is still in the mother's womb.

Another huge advance in preventing infant death from hemolytic disease of the newborn was the initiation of testing the expectant mother early in pregnancy for the Rh factor. If a woman is Rh negative, and her husband and the developing fetus are Rh positive she may develop an antibody to the antigen. Once developed, the mother retains this antibody for life, and in subsequent pregnancies her babies may die of the hemolytic disease. Now such a mother may be immunized against the disease. This knowledge has dramatically reduced mortality from it. This potential and the means of preventing it emphasizes the importance of early prenatal care.

Another major development in recent years, in the care of premature babies, has been the establishment of Neonatal Intensive Care Centers. Most of these babies were born to mothers who had not received adequate prenatal care. The cost of care of one of these "premies" in such a center averages $20,000.

Dr. Martin L. Cohen, medical Director of the Center at the Children's

Hospital in San Diego reported in 1983, that in unusual cases* costs can be tremendous. Of five infants with chronic lung disease, four were "premies" weighing less than 2.2 pounds. The accumulated costs for care exceeded $2.5 million dollars! The disheartening development was that three of these five babies expired before they reached the age of one year. This poses a problem of cost effectiveness of the limited health dollar. The fact remains, however, that refinements in care and development of centers such as these continue to reduce neonatal and infant mortalities.

Another important development that influenced the health of babies and children occurred early in the twentieth century. Some physicians with a particular interest in babies and children began to limit their practices to the care of this age group. These doctors were the first pediatricians. In the Pacific Northwest, Dr. J. B. Bilderback was considered to be the Father of Pediatrics in that area. That specialty of medicine along with many others, including obstetrics, grew. Today we have sub-specialties in pediatrics and other specialty practices.

Women began to realize the value of having their babies checked monthly during the first year of life and to obtain immunizations, advice on feeding, and to discover any abnormalities that the infant might have. This was in addition to care which the baby received if it became ill. The frequency of illness dropped as better preventive care was provided.

As health departments were developed they established well-baby and well-child clinics or Conferences. These primarily served families who could not afford to take their children to a private physician, but any child was welcomed. In these clinics the mother was given the opportunity to ask questions about the child, its health, and development. The child was given a thorough physical examination and checked on developments. Any abnormalities found were explained by the physician or nurse, and the mother was referred to her own physician for any corrective care. Advice on nutrition and general care was given. Immunizations, as indicated, were offered.

To illustrate the value of such examinations, I remember an occurrence while conducting a Well-Baby Clinic in Gold Beach, Oregon, in the early forties. Because of the shortage of physicians, I traveled over the entire state conducting Infant and Well-Child Clinics in many communities. On examining one of the babies I positioned the infant's legs together as it

---

*1% in the San Diego Center.

lay, as most physicians do, undressed, on its back on the examining table. I had done this thousands of times on other babies as part of the examination, without finding anything unusual, except in cases of a known abnormality. In this particular baby, the right leg seemed to be about one half inch shorter than the left. I re-positioned the baby to be certain of the finding. Then I measured both legs from the hip to the ankle and, confirmed that one leg was shorter than the other. Not wanting to excite the mother, I asked if she had noticed any difference in the lengths of the legs. She had not. I reassured her, and told her that it would be best to have the baby checked further by her own doctor. She asked me to call him. At that time there was only one physician in Gold Beach, Dr. Cartwright. As I knew him quite well, I called him and explained the findings and suggested that he might want to get an x-ray of the hips. He did this. The X-ray revealed a congenital dislocation of the hip. The family was referred to Crippled Children's Services. Orthopedic surgeons recommended surgical correction. After the correction, the baby developed without any evidence of the earlier abnormality. Checking the length of infants' legs thousands of times without finding a previously unrecognized abnormality was rewarded by finding this one case. If the surgery had not been performed before the baby reached the age of one year, deformity, abnormal growth, and handicapping would have occurred.

Abnormalities of the heart, hernias, squints, hearing, and vision problems, skin defects, and many other conditions were found in this preventive type of health care both in private physicians' offices and in health department clinics. As a result of immunizations, improved nutrition, and correction of abnormalities, newborn's chances of living to the age of one year rose dramatically. In 1880, about one hundred twenty-five babies out of every thousand, died before the age of one year, and by 1985, the infant mortality rate was reduced to approximately ten per thousand live births, a reduction of over 92%! The major problem remaining was that of higher infant mortality in certain ethnic groups, particularly in African Americans. The rate in this group is approximately twenty per thousand live births. In contrast, at the same time in Wyoming, the state having the lowest infant mortality in the United States, only seven infants of every thousand died before the age of one year.

Pre-schoolers in the mid part of this century were the forgotten children. Infants were being seen by pediatricians, family physicians, or health departments. Too often however, at the age of one, either another baby arrived that took priority, or the mother thought that the child only needed to be seen by a physician if it became ill. This was unfortunate as it is during these pre-school years that detection of eye, hearing, and other defects, developmental, and nutritional is vital. If defects are not detected and corrected in these pre-school years, damage often is irreparable.

In recent years pre-schoolers and kindergarten children have received considerable attention, particularly in programs like Operation Headstart. Unfortunately, children in every community of this country have not had the benefit of the program, and often inadequate staff have been unable to assure all of the care that these children need. Presently, only half of those children who should be getting this care are receiving it. Finding those in need of the service is as important as giving it!

The school-age child has generally fared better. The need to provide adequate health services for them has been recognized for decades. As early as 1900, in a few areas, some school children were being given physical examinations and concern was being expressed about the health of this age group. In an editorial appearing in the Journal of the American Medical Association in 1905, the editor wrote, "every autumn, at the beginning of the school year, it seems advisable to call attention to the fact that one of the most important features in success in school work is that the child be in normal health. It is absurd to expect the child in poor health to succeed in its studies like normal children, or even that it shall do itself justice in the trying process of development of its faculties." The editor cited a report of the Department of Health of New York on examination of 13,941 children in metropolitan schools. Of these 6,294, just under half, required medical attention. 1,092, were so poorly nourished that they required "special care on this score." In addition, it was found that 3,219 children were suffering from defective vision and 460 children had defective hearing. "Children laboring from notable defects of the most important faculties used in modern educational methods cannot be expected to keep up with other children. Many of the children considered by teachers as dull, were found to be suffering from either a defect of vision, or of hearing, for which no correction had been made. Of these children, 1,623 had breathing defects, 'mouth breathers', so much retarded by this physical abnormality that it is not surprising to find that most of these children were considered to be dull. They will continue to be backward until relieved of their serious respiratory handicap."

Over 2,300 children were suffering from enlargement of the cervical glands, "Most of these cases are doubtless tuberculosis in nature." The editor concluded, "In other words, this careful examination of school children has given valuable material not only for the educator, but also for all those who are interested in the great work of the prevention of disease."* The editor pointed out that these studies were made in poorer districts of the city, but care was taken to avoid the worst quarters, slums, "so that the results obtained might be of average value for comparative purposes." Again, I would emphasize that his editorial was written in 1905.

This erudite analysis relating health of the school aged child to his/her education is just as applicable today as it was then. Since 1905, much attention has been given to health of school children and to providing services for them. Many schools require school health examinations for entering students, either by private physicians or health departments where they exist and have the personnel to do them. Much attention also has been given to testing vision and hearing and dental health. Larger school systems have established school health programs in the schools. Others have given financial support to health departments to provide health services in the schools. Most of these programs are inadequately financed. When health examinations or inspections are made and abnormalities are found, often there is insufficient staff to visit the child's home and to explain to the parents the nature of the health problem and to assist in obtaining necessary care. In many communities, particularly in rural areas, because of budget deficiencies and lack of health personnel, school children receive very little in the way of preventive health services other than what the teacher can provide.

High school students often fail to receive such service. Some of the better schools have established a health service center where students can go for counseling on health problems, drugs, psychological, and physical problems, and in some instances receive a pre-graduation physical examination. Health departments often are utilized to provide this service.

Although school health services and the health of school children have improved greatly, there are still many deficiencies. As explained in other areas of this book, adequate financial support of protective, preventive health service for every community has never been provided. Teachers responsible for classroom education often cannot devote the needed time to health-related activities. With increasing limitations on school and health

---

*Editorial: JAMA. 1905.

department expenditures, school nurse positions are being abolished, as are many nurse positions in health departments. This materially reduces health services for children in schools, and equally important for them during the many hours they are not in school.

Many national organizations including the American School Health Association, American Public Health Association, American Medical Association, and Parent Teacher Associations have expressed their concern and have supported health programs for children. The value of these programs, many of them in demonstrations, have been well established.

Unfortunately, preventive health services for children not only are inadequate in reaching all children, but they have been so fragmented that much waste and inefficiency has resulted.

9. Mental Health Services

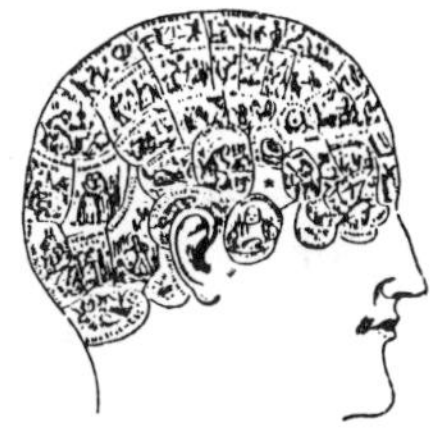

We have frequently referred to the emotional and mental influences on health. The relationship of stress to asthma, hay fever, peptic ulcer, headaches, and certain skin manifestations has been recognized for years and studied as psychosomatic medicine. More recently it has been noted that many other illnesses including high blood pressure and heart disease are closely associated with, although not necessarily caused by, emotional disorders.

Acceptance of psychological elements of disease is relatively recent. Many physicians and a large segment of the public still do not recognize the importance of this aspect of medicine. A glimpse of the development of mental health services in our society is interesting as background for our consideration of current mental health services.

In reviewing this development we should consider the medical concepts and treatments as they existed prior to this century. This will bring out clearly the tremendous progress that has been made in the mental health field in the past one hundred years. In medieval times, mentally ill persons were considered as being bewitched and possessed by demons. Many were banished or thrown into dungeons and put into chains, further terrorizing them. In the mid-sixteenth century, John Weyer was the first to recognize that these people were not possessed by demons but were suffering from mental illness.

By the mid-nineteenth century attitudes were changing slightly. Some of the deranged were allowed to wander aimlessly or were cared for in shrines, often maintained by monks, or were detained in asylums. In those families that had the means and facilities the unfortunate individual "under a spell" whose behavior was queer was often locked in a room or closeted. The primary objective was to separate these "deranged" from society and to disregard the wanderers. Medical diagnosis and treatment were unknown.

After 1900, we begin to see recognition of various kinds of disturbed people. Asylums were being transformed from detention centers to institutions for care of the chronic mentally ill and the mentally retarded. Hospitals were established for treatment of these patients. Attitudes toward mentally ill persons became one of pity with an element of compassion for these "poor creatures." They still carried the labels of "mad", "crazy", "deranged", "lunatics", or "insane'. Considerations however, were becoming more scientific, turning away from the mystic and punishment approach.

About this time, Sigmund Freud, in his studies in Paris and Vienna contributed a gigantic step forward in this evolutionary process of diagnosing and caring for the mentally ill. He attacked what had been termed hysteria, on a psychological basis. Analysis of the cause of hysteria, through hypnosis, was resulting in cures. Freud, for the first time, recognized the existence of an unconscious activity of the brain and its influence on the conscious mind. He established a concept of the influence of "infantile sexuality", the effects of repression, the Oedipus Conflict, repression of hostilities, and fears related to parents and infantile experiences. He founded the school of Psychoanalysis recognized by the first International Congress of psychoanalysis held in 1908.

Different kinds of mental illness were recognized more frequently and better described at that time, including schizophrenia, manic depressive psychosis, anxiety hysteria, paresis, toxic insanity, organic brain disease, epileptic insanity, paranoia, paralysis of the insane, neurosis, and neurasthenia.

These developments influenced programs in the United States. Many so-called "queers", or "mad" persons were still locked in their rooms. They were family skeletons, individuals that families never spoke of, that they tried to hide, and that they were ashamed of, or embarrassed about. Efforts were being made however, to get them out of the closets.

Between 1890 and 1922, many states enacted Lunacy Acts, recognizing the mentally ill and the need for more humane care. Financial responsibility was being transferred from private resources, church organizations, philanthropists, and organizations interested in the mentally ill, to the government. Medical schools began to include the teaching of psychiatry in their curricula in the late twenties and early thirties. Asylums or sanctuaries for care of the insane had been established, usually by states. These new institutions were generally under medical supervision. They often were composed of large dormitory-like buildings with many wards, dining rooms, treatment and examining rooms. Some cared for the mentally ill, others for the mentally retarded.*

I vividly remember my first visit to a state hospital in Oregon in 1928. I was taking a course in Psychology at the University of Oregon. Our class of about seventy-five students spent an afternoon at the state hospital visiting wards and listening to staff presentations, seeing individual patients, and discussing their problems. In going through the wards, I was impressed with the patients' near-normal appearance and the acceptability of their behavior. The only abnormality seemed to be in wards in which individuals were sitting around, apathetic and scarcely aware of our presence. Some persons seemed to be very despondent.

I particularly recollect two cases that were presented to us. One was an affable, jovial-appearing, rather obese woman about thirty years of age. As she entered the room, we were introduced as a college class. She said, "Oh, I see some of you are wearing sorority pins. Well, I'm a sorority girl, too. See my pin?" She displayed a huge safety pin attached to the lapel of her blouse. Then, she proceeded to tell us how she had just broken up a fight between two patients in her ward and she said, "Believe me I can do it, too! I had to sit on one of them, but I sure stopped that fight!" She continued a stream of chatter during the five to ten minutes that she was with us. We were told, as we had surmised, that she was in the manic phase of a manic-depressive psychosis.

The other patient was a man who, after being introduced and asked a few questions, began to tell us of the millions he had in the bank, the large ranch that he owned, the Cadillacs, Stanley Steamers, and Mack trucks that he operated, and of the big parties that he gave. These were fantasies but he seemed happy in them. He was suffering from paresis, resulting from infection with syphilis and destruction of his brain.

As I have mentioned in the chapter on STD, 10% or more of all patients in mental hospitals, at that time, were there due to paresis. Until the early fifties, new state hospitals were being constructed, and others expanded as more individuals with mental illnesses surfaced. It was at this time that new approaches were being taken on a trial basis, to remove selected patients from the hospital, and to care for them in the community,

*Mental retardation is usually a congenital condition, low I.Q. Mental illness is an abnormal functioning of the brain, usually in an individual with a normal or elevated I.Q.

assuring them of good psychiatric, nursing, and social care. Results were encouraging. In the fifties, at one of our State and Territorial Health Officers meetings with the Surgeon General of the USPHS, it was predicted that within a few years the need for large state hospitals would be markedly decreased as most mentally ill patients would be taken care of in their own communities. This prediction proved to be an accurate one and many mental hospitals and wards were closed in the sixties and seventies. Unfortunately, many communities without adequate public health services were not prepared to care for these patients as they were discharged. Too often, many of them ended up as part of the homeless population.

In this new era of mental health with the emphasis on treatment, rather than detention, better diagnoses were made and new treatments were tried. Psychoanalysis was used by some psychiatrists, a relatively new specialty in medicine. Treatment by psychoanalysis required at least two years and was not very applicable in a large state institution. Sedation of the patient was commonly used. In severe cases, in patients who required restraints in straight-jackets, shock therapy, and rarely lobotomy, (surgical destruction of a portion of the brain), were tried if the patient was not responding to conservative treatment. It was somewhat traumatic to witness shock therapy as given then, but it often brought otherwise hopelessly demented individuals back to reality and susceptibility to counseling and other treatment, especially patients with profound depression and involutional melancholia. As given today, shock therapy is far less traumatic but still successful in severe cases where other therapy has failed.

Potential violence of severely psychotic patients was impressed on my memory by an incident in a recently completed private general hospital built in Oregon in the mid-fifties. With the trend to admit mental patients to general hospitals, a few rooms had been reserved for mental patients and one room for violent cases. Safeguards had been taken to protect the patient. Toilet facilities were specially designed to prevent destruction and only a simple bunk bed was provided in the room. The first violent patient admitted tore the lavatory off the wall, pulled the electric outlets with wiring attached from the walls, demolished the bed and damaged the walls. It appeared as if a tornado had hit the room. Although I did not see the patient, he must have had tremendous strength.

In the late sixties, a movie entitled, "One Flew Over The Cuckoo's Nest", was shown across the country. It quite accurately depicted conditions as they had been some twenty years earlier. The movie was widely acclaimed. Unfortunately, the fact that the movie showed conditions existing twenty years earlier was not brought out in the film.*

The introduction of tranquilizing drugs was very helpful. These calmed agitated patients so that the therapist could communicate with them, generally with excellent results. One of the first of these drugs was Thorazine. Librium, Valium, and other drugs were used to combat anxiety. Thus, in the early fifties, treatment of mental illness began with chemicals supplementing psychiatric counseling, largely eliminating the need for shock therapy and similar treatments. The introduction of Lithium in the treatment of manic depressive patients represented another major advance in chemotherapy and the use of psychotropic drugs. In recent years, other useful drugs were being found by neurophysiologists, and neuropharmaceutical researchers. In addition to Lithium, drugs such as Parnate, Tofranil, and Xanax were discovered to be effective in many types of depression. The two phenothiazines, Compazine, Mellaril, in addition to Thorazine, were found to be useful in treating psychotic patients.

One of the most exciting discoveries was that of endomorphin. This is a substance occurring naturally in the brain. Its action was found to be similar to that of morphine, in sedating and in relieving pain. Better understanding of the production and control of this substance in the body promises further advances in treatment of mental disorders.

Introduction of cognitive therapy, substituting positive thinking for negative thoughts, was introduced. Group therapy, therapy involving psychiatrists, psychologists, especially trained psychiatric nurses, psychiatric social workers, and technicians as a team was introduced. Occupational therapists, physical therapists, and even attendants on the wards became members or the team in this successful cooperative approach.

These teams can have ingenious ideas. At one hospital they were dealing with a manic and another patient in depression. For occupational therapy, some patients mowed lawns. They were huge. The manic wanted to run with the hand-pushed, non-power lawn mower. He tired rapidly and couldn't mow evenly. The depressed patient just couldn't get the mower going. The staff paired the two and the results were great.

Regrettably, most of the large state hospitals had inadequate numbers of staff, particularly medical, to properly care for all of the patients. Many

---

*Dr. Dean K. Brooks, Director of the Oregon State Hospital, where much of the movie was filmed, played one of the key roles.

being committed to these hospitals were elderly, somewhat senile patients who in earlier years had been relegated to country poor farms. In many of the hospitals this type of patient often did little more than vegetate.

The most dramatic reduction in mental illness and in the admissions to state hospitals was, at first, the result of treatment of syphilis with "606", arsphenamine, neo-arsphenamine and bismuth. Later, beginning in the forties, penicillin therapy was introduced. It was very effective and replaced "606" therapy. As mentioned earlier, paresis, syphilitic infection of the brain which can develop as a late stage of syphilis, now rarely occurred and the numbers of such patients in state hospitals rapidly dropped. Early diagnosis and treatment of persons with syphilis represented a major preventive measure for this type of mental illness.

In the late forties and fifties, local communities were awakening to the needs of the mentally ill. In addition they were becoming aware of the need to promote good mental health, to avoid alcoholism, drug abuse, suicides, and other behavioral problems. Community mental health programs were being established in a few areas. One of the outstanding local programs was that established in St. Louis, Missouri. It was a truly cooperative program centered in the county health department where Dr. Herbert R. Domke, Commissioner of Health, established a mental health division in his department. St. Louis schools, Mental Health association of St. Louis, Parent Teacher Associations, and many other groups cooperated to make this program an outstanding success. Margaret C.L. Gildea, M.D., served as the psychiatrist consultant to the project. Initiated about 1947, it was continued for many years and received national recognition. The emphasis here was on prevention, working with children, parents, and schools. Groups of parents were assisted in child-rearing through a series of parent conferences and discussions. To utilize better the limited numbers of psychiatric personnel available, the professionals served as consultants and the parents with leadership abilities led the group discussions. This program became very popular over a period of many years, involving a large portion of the young parents of the county. Supplementing this was a program of consultation with teachers, public health nurses, school nurses, and parents, using psychiatrists, psychologists, and other mental health personnel to demonstrate techniques of helping the children with emotional or other behavioral problems. Children with more serious problems were seen in child guidance clinics but these clinics were used to demonstrate to teachers and parents the methods and techniques of helping children, in order that parents and teachers might utilize these techniques. This was preferable to building large child guidance clinic caseloads. The program, with community response, illustrated how community interest in mental health was increasing.

I promoted a similar demonstration project with a small church group in Oregon. Our Child Psychiatrist and Psychiatric Social Service Worker served as consultants to a group of ten married couples, either expecting babies or having children of various ages, including teenagers. Twelve sessions were held, one each week for about two hours. The professional staff met with the group the first and last sessions and made themselves available as needed for others. Characteristic of newborn, infants, two year olds, three and four year olds, pre-schoolers, early elementary school students, junior high, and high school students were discussed.

One of the couples was made responsible for reading up on a particular age group, showing a film, and initiating the discussion on that group. A series of films depicting age characteristics such as the "terrible twos", the "trusting threes", and the "fearsome fours" were shown. Problems being encountered and introduced by one couple were discussed. Other parents that had had similar problems related their experiences. This free exchange between parents, showing the films, and sharing the literature gave parents more confidence and understanding in parenting. Young couples were enthusiastic in their praise of the series and the helpfulness to them. The pastor of the church told me that one of the husbands was an alcoholic. As a result of the discussions, he obtained professional help and overcame his problem. In the case of another couple, the "wife wore the pants" in the family, dominating its activities. After the series she mended her ways, permitting the somewhat docile husband to assume an equal role in family management. These were by-products of the series. The couples, as a whole, benefited and were better able to understand their children, to communicate with them, to handle problems and to know that resources were available to help in situations in which they did not feel competent.

The group of couples was unanimous in recommending additional series for other parents. Some offered to help or even lead other groups. Unfortunately, our mental health staff of two had responsibilities for statewide Child Guidance programs and were unable to give the necessary time to help other young parents with a similar series. It was a disappointment to me and to the church as well, that this type of program could not be continued and extended.

In Oregon during the fifties and sixties, as a result of community interest and with the support of the state legislature, Child Guidance Clinics were established in Portland by the University of Oregon Medical School staff and in the rest of the state by a team composed of Child Psychiatrist, Dr. John Waterman, and his wife, Minnie waterman, a Psychiatirc Social Worker. We were fortunate in having this husband and wife team as much travel was required over the state of Oregon, encompassing about 120,000 square miles.

This program was helping to meet the needs of children, but a major deficiency in the state hospital program (primarily for adults) was recognized. There was little communication between the hospital staff and local health departments. Cases were not being referred for Health Department staff nurses to visit the families of patients, advise the hospital staff of home conditions prior to patient discharge, and to follow-up on patients, assisting them to readjust in the community. The hospital staff believed that the local health department staff was not qualified to assist in dealing with patients and that confidentiality would be threatened.

An incident occurred that convinced state hospital staff otherwise. A young mother from a southern Oregon county had been hospitalized for a number of months. At the time of her discharge, no inquiry was made in the community regarding her family nor was there any attempt to prepare her family for her return home. When she reached home, she found that her husband had deserted her and that her children had been placed in a foster home. The shock was too great for her. She committed suicide. Review of this case emphasized the need for continuing communication between the state hospitals and the community before, during, and after hospitalization.

Arrangements were made for a week of orientation at the state hospital for selected local health department public health nurses who would be involved in this type of visitation. The orientation proved to be two-way, with not only the public health nurses learning about hospital care and needs in community follow-up, but the hospital staff learning about the abilities of the public nurses and of the resources available in the community. Although most health departments did not have sufficient staff to follow all discharged patients and many counties did not have health departments, the limited program was successful and represented another step forward in improving care of mental patients.

Other states were establishing similar community mental health programs assisted with funds provided through a national mental health act. North Carolina, Kansas, Georgia, and California were among those recognized for their early pioneering programs. California enacted a Short-Doyle Act which required the majority of counties of the state, the more populous ones, to establish county-wide community mental health programs. These included provision of local diagnostic, and treatment clinics, emergency services for psychiatric patients and drug abusers, short term hospitalization, home visitation, and promotion of good mental health. We will discuss one California program in more detail, subsequently. These were, and still are, proving to be very successful. The Act provided for local administration and involvement of the community through establishment of an advisory committee with most of the members being consumers. Ninety percent of the funds were provided by the state.

As community mental health programs developed, consideration was given to alternatives to state hospital care. Many reasons for limiting growth of state hospitals and for reducing the numbers of patients kept in them were found. High cost of care was a major factor. In California, local Boards appreciated cost because under the Short-Doyle program, the counties were required to pay for ten percent of the cost of state hospital care. Even the ten percent cost to the county brought the realization that patient care in a state facility still costs a substantial amount of money. Prior to the Short-Doyle program, the state bore the entire expense. More important reasons were recognition of the need for continuity of care, and of the shock to a patient in being committed and being sent away from home and family to a distant hospital. It was further realized that there was a subsequent shock to the patient upon discharge from the hospital with the need to adjust to home and local community life after having lived in a sheltered hospital setting. These were good reasons to provide treatment in the community as an alternative to state hospital care. As a result, many state hospitals were closed.

It was recognized that for some patients who did not respond to known treatment and who could not cope with conditions outside of the hospital, and for the criminally insane, some state hospitals must be retained and be adequately staffed.

Controversy developed as to the wisdom of releasing so many patients to the community without provision for adequate follow-up and treatment. Unfortunately, in too many areas, provision for good community care was not made. My experience in actually visiting patients in some state hospitals and seeing their condition, compared to individuals who did receive good follow-up care in the community, convinced me that in most instances, good community care was preferable to the care provided in large state institutions. Many who criticize the inadequacy of community care and who suggest return to the state hospitalization plan, forget or never saw conditions as they were when the large portion of mentally ill persons were "shipped off" to state hospitals. They see only the relatively few who have ended up as part of the homeless. Rather than return these patients to state hospitals, critics should support adequately financed, well administered community mental health services and care.

Commitment procedures also were changed requiring in most instances, local evaluation for a period of seventy-two hours or more to determine if a commitment was needed.

To illustrate the type of community mental health program that I have referred to, we might look at a program developed in the early seventies in Riverside, one of California's rapidly growing counties, with a population of over 200,000. This county encompasses an area of over 8,000 square miles, from fifty miles east of Los Angeles to the Arizona border. This conservative county had little in the way of government local mental health facilities. The Riverside General Hospital, (county sponsored), had fewer than forty beds for psychiatric patients, to serve the entire county. Riverside had a number of excellent private psychiatrists and a privately operated psychiatric clinic. Palm springs, Hemet, and Indio had limited psychiatric resources.

In 1969, Riverside and San Bernadino counties, the last in the state to develop community mental health programs under the Short-Doyle Act, were mandated by state legislation to develop community mental health services. There was little interest on the part of Riverside General Hospital staff or other county departments, in assuming responsibility for developing this new program. The County Administrative Officer, CAO, was reluctant to establish a new department to administer the program. As recently appointed Director of Health, having a long-term interest in mental health, and knowing that many studies had shown that public health and mental health could most effectively be administered, and conducted in one department, I volunteered to assume responsibility for developing the new Mental Health Program.

The County Board of Supervisors quickly accepted the offer. It was a big task. Fortunately, state consultation and financial assistance simplified the problem, but it was still difficult to plan needed programs, to set priorities, to justify and to obtain the necessary ten percent matching funds from the County. A conservative CAO was reluctant to recommend requests for adequate needed funds but given a good explanation, and with the support of a Mental Health Advisory Board, a cooperative Board of Supervisors approved our requests, occasionally over the objections of the CAO.

The Mental Health Advisory Board was chaired by a dynamic community leader, Erna Poliak, who, along with others on the Board, gave a great deal of time to assist in planning and developing the program. With the establishment of plans, priorities, (which we will describe) and with the availability of funds, staff was now needed to implement the plans. Recruiting became a formidable task. We finally arranged to employ an able Child Psychiatrist, Dr. Richard Griffin, as chief of the Mental Health Division. We shared his services with Loma Linda Medical School. After a lengthy search, we recruited one of the very scarce psychiatric nurses trained in public health. Psychologists, psychiatric social workers, essential secretarial assistance and administrative staff were employed.

Outpatient clinics were established at the Health Department, at Riverside General Hospital, and in various centers in the county. This service was supplemented through a contract with a private psychiatric clinic, to provide outpatient clinic service on a fee basis paid for by the county. The latter, the first arrangement of this kind in California under the Short-Doyle program, was helpful in getting the program started. Hospitals in the county became interested in providing psychiatric care. With federal assistance, the Hemet Hospital built an addition for mental health care. It was a model unit, more like a first class hotel than what most of us had visualized a psychiatric hospital unit to be. We contracted with this hospital to provide inpatient and outpatient care for the eastern portion of Riverside County to supplement that provided by the Riverside General Hospital. In the late seventies, the Desert Hospital, a private hospital in Palm Springs, with a federal grant, built an addition which eventually would provide as many as one hundred beds for psychiatric patients. Initially, it cared for about twenty patients. As the program expanded, services, in cooperation with the schools, were provided for school children with emotional problems. Authorized by special state legislation, methadone programs were established for heroin addicts and special programs were also established for alcoholics. By 1974, almost five hundred former heroin addicts, many of whom told us of shoplifting and burglarizing homes to maintain their expensive addictions, were under treatment. Hotlines were established where persons with emotional problems, including those with suicidal tendencies, drug addicts, and alcohol addicts could call to get emergency assistance, advice or emotional support.

Recognizing the need to provide good community care as an alternative to hospitalization, arrangements were made for care of patients at nursing or custodial care homes, or in their own homes. To assure good psychiatric treatment, teams of psychiatrists, psychiatric social service workers, and nurses visited the patients in the homes regularly, sometimes as often as once a week. It was very gratifying to see the response of these patients to the freedom and home surroundings. Many that I had seen in wards of state hospitals merely sitting around day after day with little activity or interest in their surroundings, now were up and about and often helping with simple tasks in and about the home. Yes, there were failures, but the teams detected these early and initiated more intense treatment, occassionally re-hospitalization was required.

Another innovation was establishing an emergency center for diagnosis and treatment of emotionally disturbed persons. A psychiatrist, present or on call, and staff were available to see an individual thought to need hospitalization because of psychiatric symptoms, at any hour, day or night. Diagnosis could be made and treatment started immediately or if necessary, the patient could be kept under observation for a few hours, for diagnosis and treatment. Often, with prompt treatment, the individual could be returned to his or her home, without the added complications and cost of hospitalization.

With these resources available, the number of patients from Riverside County in the State Hospitals was reduced from about four hundred and fifty in 1969, to approximately fifty in 1974. The cost of good community care was no greater, and in many instances less than care in the State Hospitals. Mental health programs of this kind were established not only in the state of California but in most parts of the United States.

In the mid-seventies, congress enacted legislation to provide special mental health programs for poverty areas. Plans for such projects were approved and Mental Health Centers were established in many parts of the country. Advisory Boards composed of community leaders were established to assist in administration of these special programs. Riverside County established one in the Palm Springs area, the Desert Community Mental Health Center.

Administration was complex as the Director of the program was responsible to an Advisory Board of almost twenty community members, the Director of the Riverside County Health and Mental Health Department and to the Riverside County Board of Supervisors. These Centers brought Mental Health Services to population groups most difficult to serve. Federal funds for these special projects helped to assure their success.

We have discussed, but only slightly, the developments in diagnosis and treatment of specific mental diseases and the contributions of the private sector in this development of mental health services. These, have been extensive. Diagnosis has become more precise and new treatments have been very effective.

What goes on behind the door of the psychiatrist's consultation room? For years we heard of his or her couch. This was primarily a symbol of the need for the patient to relax. As stated earlier, psychoanalysis required at least two years of sessions to determine the basis for the patient's conduct. For a variety of reasons, one being cost, and another the time required, this approach is not as frequently used as it was in earlier years. Once communication is established with a patient, more direct means of determining the cause and treating it are now used. Videotapes of patients are proving to be helpful as an aid in helping them understand themselves.

One way mirrors that permit observation, particularly of troubled children, are helpful in diagnosis. I have seen a distraught child alone in a room with finger paints, display many kinds of feelings. Not realizing that he or she is being observed, and being alone, innermost feelings are often portrayed with use of paints. Sometimes the room suffers as a result. The objective is to learn what those inner feelings are. Observation by staff members, particularly in hospital settings, often contribute a great deal to understanding and helping the patient.

In caring for patients in hospitals, much consideration has been given to the amount of freedom that can be permitted. For a time the hope was that locks on doors of psychiatric units in hospitals could be abolished. Patients would be free to leave at any time. There would be no feeling of restraint. For many patients this was helpful. For some however, it was not realistic since patients would wander away, jeopardizing themselves and sometimes others. In many hospitals today, much freedom is given in a unit but the entrance and the exit to the unit is usually limited.

Recreational and occupational therapy are great adjuncts to treatment. Small kitchen and dining room facilities are often available to the patients to enhance their feeling of independence. Group therapy, giving patients the opportunity of helping each other often supports the psychiatric treatment.

Judicious use of tranquilizers, anti-depressants, and other drugs, depending on the individual needs of a patient, are very effective. We have mentioned limited use of shock therapy and hypnosis.

Child psychiatry has become an important segment of the field. Determining the basis for a child's problem and resolving it in cooperation with the parents has been successful. Early recognition of the need for psychiatric consultation, both for children, teenagers, and adults, is as important as recognizing the early signs and symptoms of cancer. The lives of many suicidal persons could have been saved if only their suggestive comments had been taken seriously.

Obviously, private psychiatrists, psychiatric staff, clinics, and hospitals, in cooperation with government facilities are making a major contribution to better community mental health.

The importance of this is emphasized when we recognize that it was estimated in the fifties that ten percent of our population was either in, had been, or would be, in a mental institution. In addition, millions of persons suffered from depression, anxiety, and phobias which prevented the full enjoyment of life. Although there are still deficiencies in service and controversies over what the best type of care for the mentally ill actually should be, tremendous progress has been made. The crisis in care is due to fragmentation and inadequate funding of community mental health services.

In considering the mental health problems for the community the developmentally retarded were not forgotten. Early in the century as we have mentioned, state facilities were provided for the care of the mentally retarded. President John F. Kennedy and his wife had a major interest in helping these handicapped persons. Stimulated by their interest, national legislation was enacted and federal financial assistance became available to aid in development of better programs for them. Community attitudes changed. Seldom were the words, "imbecile", "moron", "idiot" or "Mongolian idiot" used. New, more appropriate terminology such as "developmentally retarded" and "Down's Syndrome" reflect new attitudes and with them improved help for the retarded. Special homes and schools for the retarded were developed in communities. Fewer children were sent to state facilities and some of those in state facilities were transferred to local community facilities.

Again, a difference of opinion existed as to whether state facilities, local facilities, or the individuals own home was best. Actually there was, and is, need for all three. Each individual and his or her family circumstances must be considered. Many severely retarded persons do better in state facilities where they can associate with others having similar levels of disability. In some families, or where the individual does not have a family, provision for suitable non-institutional care is not always possible.

There are those who think that the occupants of state facilities are unhappy. On the contrary, I have seen children in such facilities quite happy as they do not have to compete and they are not looked down on or mocked by some of their classmates. I remember seeing resident couples on the grounds of a state facility, joyfully walking hand-in-hand, on their way to the cafeteria. Others, in classrooms or at play appeared to be enjoying themselves. Institutional staff often with the assistance of volunteers, have helped numerous retardates achieve their maximum potential. Many handicapped children whose parents can give the necessary care, and express their love for their children without neglecting other children in the family, develop and achieve better than they would in a large facility such as a state institution. Loving parents with assistance from special teachers, psychologists, social workers, and other professional staff have accomplished incredible results in promoting development and reducing dependence of the handicapped on others. Special schools and sheltered living have been invaluable.

I remember visiting one of the special schools and seeing some of the children and the remarkable progress they were making. One little girl, about eight years of age, had been fed, clothed, and kept clean by a loving mother who had taken care of the child twenty-four hours a day for the child's entire life. What patience. The child could not speak, feed herself, was not toilet trained, and had difficulty in walking. Staff of this special public school, after hearing of the plight of the child and of the mother, visited the home and explained the assistance that could be given through the school. Initially, the mother believed that it was not feasible to send the child to a school. She could not give her up for six to eight hours a day. Finally, she was convinced that it should be tried. A special bus picked up the little girl early in the morning, took her to the school, and returned her to her home after the days activities. Several of the staff worked with the child. After three months she was toilet trained. After another three months sufficient communication was established that the girl was able to point to her own name out of a list of several names, was able to designate the day of the month, day of the week, and the year. She was partially able to feed herself and to dress. What a change this assistance made in the life of this little girl and in the life of her family. Fortunately most of these retarded children are not as severely handicapped. Depending on the amount of retardation, with assistance, many are able to achieve productive lives. It is now being discovered that many of the developmentally retarded are more responsible and productive on some jobs than many employees.

Prevention was not neglected. Through research, education, and genetic counseling, through improved pre-natal care and better obstetrical procedures, through reduction in many of the infectious diseases, that in some cases resulted in retardation, the incidence of retardation was reduced. Unfortunately with drug abuse, teenage pregnancy, and lack of pre-natal care, this problem is increasing again. Much has been accomplished, but more needs to be done. Preventive services offer the greatest opportunity for reduction of both the problem of mental health and of mental retardation. The conquest of paresis primarily through prevention, exemplifies what the future may hold in prevention of other problems of the mind.

10. Transformation of Hospitals And Other Care Facilities

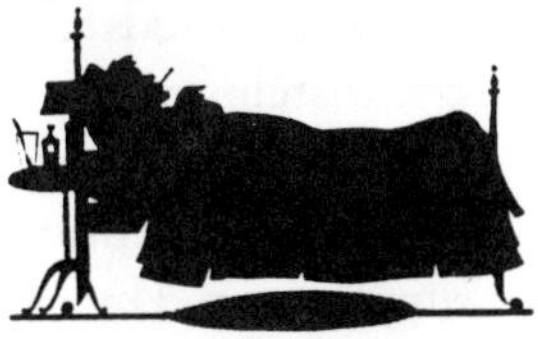

THE VERY SIGNIFICANT changes in the character of hospitals and in the quality of care given in them occurred over a period of many years. Developments in nursing homes, rehabilitation, and related facilities were also gradual. Nevertheless, the changes were dramatic. The USPHS, state and local health departments played a major role in bringing these changes about. As late as the thirties, most hospitals were rather stark-looking brick, concrete, or wooden buildings, or converted large, old residences, having limited parking; drab white, sparsely furnished rooms and wards; and had small surgeries, delivery rooms, and laboratories. Compare these with today's beautifully designed, usually spacious, air-conditioned, colorful, often carpeted, well-equipped hospitals, landscaped and with large parking areas. Today, furnishings and equipment usually include special electrically controlled positioning beds, patient monitoring equipment connected to a central nursing center, oxygen piped into the room, television, telephone, comfortable chairs, private toilet and shower facilities, and in some hospitals, live-in quarters for the patient's family adjacent to the patient's room. In addition, today's hospitals have modern surgeries with the latest scientific equipment for surgery of many kinds. Some are equipped for; open-heart surgery; organ transplants; complicated eye surgery; advanced orthopedic surgery, including joint replacements; laser beam and computer-directed surgery; as well as other very specialized procedures.

Many of today's hospitals have complex laboratories with equipment to analyze blood samples automatically and to perform other special tests. All have efficient x-ray equipment. Many have brain scanners and some have extremely expensive equipment for complete body scans. many use ultra-sound, magnetic resonance imaging, and other advanced diagnostic tools.

Nurseries provide aseptic care for newborns and generally there are special incubators, and monitoring devices for the care of premature babies.

Food is prepared in modern kitchens that often surpass in cooking, storage, and dishwashing facilities, the kitchens of some of our finest restaurants. Special diets as prescribed by the patient's physician, are meticulously prepared and served. Daily menus from which the patient may select foods most palatable to him or her, generally are available. Appropriately warm or cold appetizing foods have replaced the poor quality foods that many of the older hospitals were known to serve.

One might characterize many of our hospitals today as luxurious hotels, supplemented by room service and providing the finest kind of scientific, medical, surgical, and obstetrical services. The contrast between the hospital of the thirties and those of today is quite spectacular.

How did these changes come about? Who originally pioneered the concept of hospitals? Who sponsored and financed the building, equipping, and staffing of those initial hospitals, and who finances our modern hospitals, nursing homes, and related facilities? How successful was this planning in meeting the needs of our vast country with its rapidly growing population? These are some of the questions we will consider.

Since, in most states, there were no provisions for licensing or inspecting, very few records, and no recognized standards for structure, staffing, equipping, or service for hospitals during the first third of this century, it is difficult to describe them. In addition, there was no coordinated planning to assure that hospitals would be of appropriate size to operate efficiently and be located to best meet the needs of the public.

John Fothergill who lived in the latter part of the eighteenth century is considered to be one of the first to promote the concept of a hospital. As our country was settled and grew in population, the need for hospitals also grew. Churches or religious organizations, groups of doctors or individual physicians, and state and county governments recognized the need and either built, established, or prevailed on some philanthropist to build the early hospitals. The majority were sponsored by church groups. In many communities, physicians, either singly, or in groups, built hospitals or converted old residences into hospitals. Stately and often picturesque old homes were sometimes used.

A brief look at one of the early hospitals gives us a better idea of what they were like.

A good illustration of one built with moneys contributed by a private

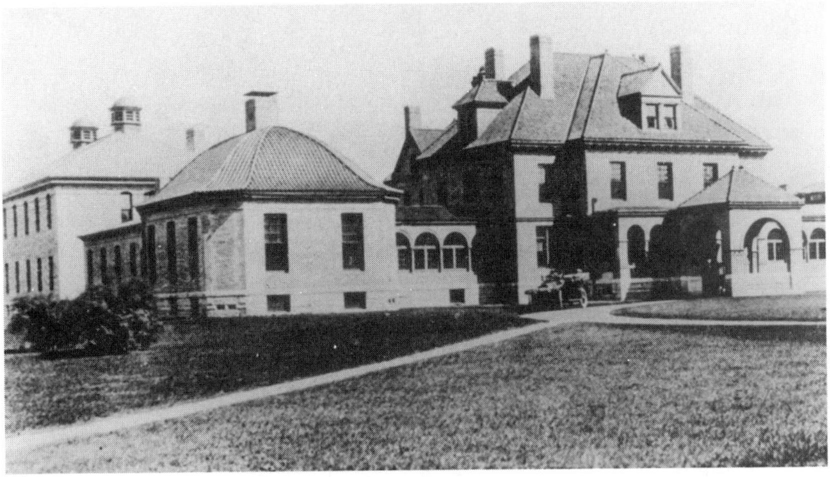

philanthropist is the Mary Hitchcock Memorial Hospital in Hanover, New Hampshire, home of Dartmouth College. It was given to the city by Mr. Hitchcock in memory of his wife. Completed in 1893, it was a three-story, forty bed hospital constructed with heavy wooden timbers and faced with yellow brick. Each room had a fireplace, the only means of heating. The water supply was provided from a huge twenty-five hundred gallon water tank on the roof. A portico at the main entrance permitted the entry of two-horse-drawn express wagons to unload patients. These were the ambulances of the day. The wagons had a ten foot flat bed. Occasionally a smaller wagon had to be used. In one instance, my one hundred year old friend, Ross Nichols, who told me about this hospital, remembers a man being brought in on a barn door, placed on the ledges of a smaller wagon. The original hospital would have seemed crude by todays standards, but it was elegant then, and it met a real community need. This particular hospital has been modernized and markedly expanded to a fine, modern facility. The original unit met community needs as they were then perceived as well as serving as the nucleus for future growth.

Governments also built some of the early hospitals. Many states built them for care of tuberculosis patients and others for care of the mentally ill. Some states built facilities for the mentally retarded, often including a small hospital section. Counties recognized a need for hospitals and built them to care for the poor and for patients with communicable diseases

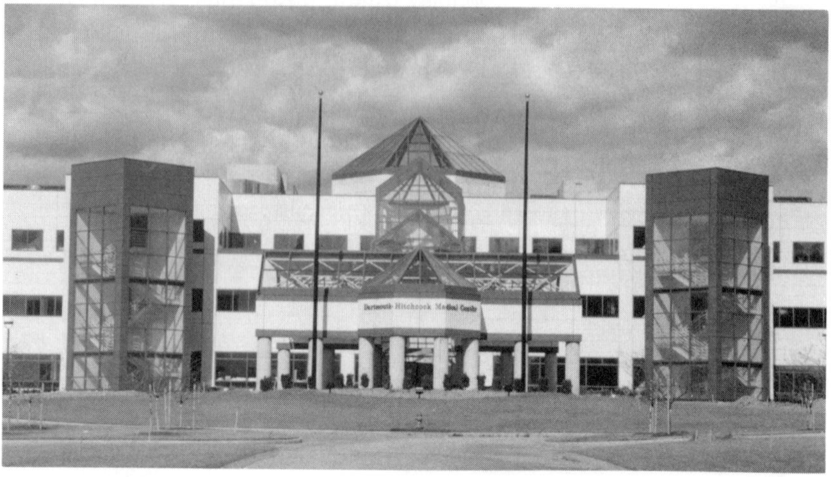

photo by Stuart Bretesman/Dartmouth College

requiring isolation. The latter hospitals, or units in county hospitals, met a need in protecting the community, but patients did not always receive the quality of care that could have been given if fear of the patient's infection had not been so great. Location of these units away from centers of medical care, and inadequacy of staffing and funding were real handicaps. Too often they were isolated, not only from the community but also from medical facilities.

Gradually, without much community planning, additional hospitals were built during the 1910's and 1920's. Many were expanded. The stock market crash of 1929, followed by the Great Depression, and then World War II, which lasted until 1945, drastically reduced previous types of financial support.

When World War II terminated, the acute need for hospitals, skilled nursing homes, and convalescent hospital facilities became critical. In 1946, Congress recognized the great deficiency in hospital and convalescent facility beds throughout the country and the urgent need for coordinated planning, establishing standards, and for supervision of the construction of such facilities. Congress also recognized the needs for funds to assist communities in building or remodeling hospitals and chronic disease facilities.

The Hill-Burton Hospital Construction Act was enacted. Congress authorized appropriations and made funds available to implement the Act.

When the program began, practically all of the states designated State

Health Departments as the agencies to administer the program. It was recognized that health departments had the kinds of professional staff, the vital statistics, and other records on hospital needs essential for good planning. They were experienced in dealing with legislatures and the public. Further, they had an established working relationship with the Public Health Service, designated as the federal agency to administer the program. Large sums of money were involved and it was recognized that there would be a great deal of competition for limited funds. Health departments had a reputation of being impartial and relatively free of "politics" and political pressures.

In 1947, many states in order to qualify for these funds, and urged by state boards of health to do so, enacted legislation which provided for the inspection and licensing of hospitals, nursing homes, and related facilities. State boards of health generally administered the licensing and the new hospital construction programs. As provided for in the federal act, legislatures established Advisory Councils on Hospital construction and on Licensing, to advise the Boards.

Obtaining state legislation was not easy. To illustrate, in Oregon, the staff of the State Board of Health had prepared a bill on licensing, and another on hospital construction, to be introduced into the legislature. The Board also included in the 1947-48 budget, provision for a modest staff of three full-time persons and some part-time assistance for these new programs. These bills were cleared with and had the endorsement of the Oregon State Medical Society, Hospital Administrators, voluntary health organizations, Senator Jack Lynch, Chairman of the public Health Committee of the Senate, and others with an interest in the proposed bills. With Senator Lynch's enthusiastic support, the bills were introduced in the Senate as "Committee bills". This gave them high priorities. There were some unforeseen complications, but these were overcome. The bills were passed, almost unanimously by both houses and were signed into law by the Governor.

These were enabling and standard setting laws, but how were they to be enforced? Limited funds had been appropriated to employ staff. Initially, only three full-time people were authorized to do all of the work required for these huge tasks. A survey of all existing hospitals and nursing homes was required. Standards and regulations for licensing needed to be prepared. An even bigger job was to develop a State Hospital plan showing the requirements for hospital and nursing home beds in the entire state and setting priorities for financial assistance to all communities based on need. As in other states, after approval by the Advisory Council, the Board and the USPHS, the Plan had to be implemented. In Oregon, this seemed like an overwhelming job for such a small staff.

We were fortunate in employing as Director of the program, an attorney, George Shiffer, who had given up a successful law practice in the midwest to move to Oregon. We also recruited an able nurse, Aura Neely, who had had considerable hospital experience. Together with a capable secretary, this staff enthusiastically undertook the work necessary to implement the program. Local Health Departments assisted in obtaining necessary data. Initially, a survey was made of the hospitals and nursing homes. We were fortunate in obtaining the assistance of Willard Stone, M.D., for four months to make the initial inspections and to evaluate buildings, equipment, and staff. Studies were conducted of the population, its distribution, numbers and location of medical, nursing, and technical personnel, the amount and kinds of industry in each community, the incidence of illness and accidents, birth and mortality rates, location of trade centers, highways, and other data bearing on hospital needs. Based on this data and the results of preliminary hearings throughout the state, a State Hospital Plan was developed. It showed existing hospitals, nursing homes, and the areas needing new or additional facilities. The goal, at that time, as established by the USPHS, was to provide four and one-half hospitals beds per thousand population. Priorities were developed based on relative needs of the various communities. The Advisory Council on Hospital Construction conducted public hearings on the plan. Some of these were quite stormy as various community leaders and hospital administrators vied to obtain top priorities for the limited federal funds. Following these hearings the Council made its recommendations to the State Board of Health.

After further hearings by the Board, appropriate changes were made in the Plan. With the Board's approval the plan was submitted to the USPHS for final approval. I have gone into some detail on procedure as it reflects a democratic process which was followed each year in revising the Plan to reflect changing conditions.

The limited federal funds were available to the states allotting one dollar of federal moneys for each two dollars provided by qualified sponsors. These were non-profit organizations or governments who would agree to meet construction and operating standards, who would care for medically indigent persons, if other resources were not available to them, who would accept patients "irrespective of race, color, or creed", and who would agree to repayment of a portion of the federal funds if the hospital or related facility was sold or converted to other use within twenty years. A few states, like California, provided one dollar of state money for each dollar of federal money available, thus reducing the sponsor's share to one third. Most states did not do this but did equally well in building hospitals, because the matching funds were raised by the communities who recognized the bed need. It did require more community involvement and support to raise the funds. This often resulted in more support for the hospital after construction. This was very important as few people realized that it costs about as much to operate a hospital for three years as it does to construct and equip it.

Professional fund raising organizations employed by the hospital sponsors, were very successful in obtaining public contributions to assist in financing these new facilities. They worked with community groups, helped them organize, and advised them on the most effective means of raising funds. The local organizations were made up of businessmen and women, some health professionals, community leaders, and other interested people. They were dedicated and gave much of their time, strictly on a voluntary basis. A group of this kind in Lebanon, Oregon, met every morning "at six", for several months, to plan and successfully complete a fund drive. Many of the members of the group contributed sizable sums of money for the project. Later, the same group continued to meet to review progress on construction, furnishing, equipping, and staffing of the new hospital. Such personal sacrifice and activity was occurring in every state. Support for hospitals came from the community, from the "grass roots." It was essential to the success of the program.

The licensing program was of real assistance to the construction program. It applied to both old and new facilities. The major objective of the licensing program was to offer consultation and help to facilities with deficiencies, in correcting them. The inadequacies could be in staffing, records, techniques, equipment, or in the physical structure of the buildings.

In addition to initial inspections by Dr. Stone, each facility was checked by the State Fire Marshall's office and was required to make any changes recommended by that office. This was a sound requirement as rather serious fire hazards, including many in state and county hospitals, were found and eliminated. In contrast to experiences in some states, not a single disastrous fire is known to have occurred in Oregon's hospitals or nursing homes. Major problems encountered included the lack of qualified nurses serving at night; over-crowding of patients, (often patients were found in beds in halls or on porches); and failure to recognize hazards or to establish proper procedures to avoid spread of infections through the hospital. Inadequacies in serving food were common. Incompleteness of physicians and nurses records on the status of patients occurred, (more commonly, the physicians!)

Another common problem encountered was that of cross-connections in plumbing. Arthur Farrell, Chief of Plumbing for the Department, checked the hospital and home facilities for adequacy of plumbing. He was recognized nationally for his pioneering efforts in focusing attention on the hazards of cross-connections. Such cross-connections of pure and polluted or drain water could be serious. Failure to install vacuum-breakers on equipment requiring them could be debilitating.* The findings of these inspections clearly confirmed one of the values of licensing hospitals.

There were relatively few nursing homes in existence anywhere in the country in 1948. There were some maternity homes. Usually the nursing homes were housed in converted private homes and were operated by well-meaning women, some of whom had training in nursing. They generally provided TLC, but in many cases they were not qualified to give medications as prescribed by the physicians. Many of the operators of these homes had very little knowledge of appropriate diets for their patients and could not recognize important new symptoms requiring a physician's attention. They were unable to provide technical nursing care for their patients. The converted old residences frequently were found to have serious fire hazards, plumbing deficiencies, inadequate kitchens and dishwashing facilities, and were not arranged to provide good quality nursing care.

The operators of some of these homes, aware of these deficiencies, and unable to correct them, closed voluntarily or converted the nursing home into a home for the aged. These homes often attempted to care for persons who really needed nursing care. It was finally agreed that the individual who could be responsible for, and who was capable of taking his or her own medications, could reside in one of these "Homes for the aged." Here again, inspections substantiated the need for licensing.

Only once in the early years of licensing programs was it necessary to seek court action to bring a Home into compliance. The outcome was surprising. A Nursing Home in a rural county was considered by our staff

*As we discussed earlier, on one occasion a cross-connection was found where the exhaust piping of a large steam sterilizer for surgical linens, instruments, and supplies, was hooked directly to a sewer without a vacuum-breaker!

to be the most deficient in Oregon at that time. Repeated warnings, official and non-official, failed to bring the home into compliance with the most basic nursing and sanitation requirements. Medications were being given without prescriptions. Records were incomplete. Diets were questionable. Patients were found with soiled linens that obviously had not been changed for hours. Inadequate staffing resulted in one nurse trying to care for the patients twenty-four hours a day, every day of the week. There were structural defects with irregular "galloping floors" and fire hazards. Litter was found inside and outside the Home. On the last inspection, a horse was found tethered to the back porch rail. Accumulated excrement made it obvious that the horse had been there for some time.

Out of concern for the patients, the operator of the Home was cited to appear before the State Board of Health. Based on the evidence, the Board denied the Nursing Home a license and gave the operator thirty days in which to meet the standards or to move the patients to other facilities. The operator appealed to the local court. Six months elapsed before the court scheduled a hearing. At the hearing the Judge asked if we would agree to a "Trial de Nova." This meant that new evidence could be presented. As our primary effort was to bring the home up to acceptable standards for care, and we wished to cooperate, we agreed. The attorney for the Home presented written testimony from former patients extolling the operator and the care they had received in the Home. Letters from local physicians explained that although there were some deficiencies, this was the only Nursing Home in the County and that it was needed. Additional evidence and a re-inspection showed that a great effort had been made to clean up the premises. The horse was gone!

Based on the new evidence, the Judge ordered the Board to issue a license. Although we had lost the case, we had accomplished our major objective of bringing the Home up to a standard where reasonably good nursing care could be given.* One cannot, and probably should not, attempt to reach standards beyond those which the residents of a community understand and support..

As modern nursing homes and convalescent facilities were built, adequately staffed and equipped, the earlier versions of Nursing Homes faded away. As newer knowledge became available standards were raised and

---

*However, the incident confirmed a conclusion reached in a court case in which the Board attempted and failed in an effort to close a hazardous restaurant in Oregon.

the rules and regulations were revised after public hearings.

The "Hospital Plan" was revised each year. We were fortunate in recruiting for our staff a young engineer, Jay Cole, to review plans, make surveys, and to assist in revisions of the "Hospital Plan". He also made inspections and consulted with the contractors to assure that the construction met our standards. Inspections revealed, and hospital administrators confirmed, the need for specialized consultation to improve maternity and infant care in hospitals. As discussed earlier, in 1951 an appropriation was obtained to employ an especially well-trained nurse in the techniques of infant and maternal care for this type of consultation. Miss Nora Lalor was recruited for the position. She visited hospitals on request, and as word of her ability spread, she was in great demand.

With this type of consultation and inspection to assure compliance with licensing standards, facilities in Oregon and throughout the country improved greatly. Hospitals were very cooperative and, given a reasonable length of time in which to improve, made many changes.

The greatest difficulty encountered was in bringing state hospitals up to standard. This was particularly true with fire safety and plumbing requirements. Many units of the state hospitals were old and corrections were expensive. Early legislatures failed to appropriate the necessary funds required, biennium after biennium. Finally, as a result of publicity and personal conferences with state officials and legislators, moneys were appropriated to make essential improvements. They finally recognized that it was not reasonable for the state to require non-governmental hospitals to meet standards and for the state to operate hospitals failing to meet the same standards.

Another important element in improving the standards of hospitals was inspection by representatives of the Joint Commission on Hospital Accreditation. This national commission, sponsored by the American Medical and Hospital Associations, as we have said, was particularly interested in qualifications of personnel and professional practices in the hospitals.

Now that we have reviewed the licensing program we should look more closely at the construction program which played an even greater role in helping states meet their hospital needs.

As an example, the initial Oregon Hospital Construction Plan, adopted in 1948, gave the highest priority for a new hospital to the area of Tillamook, Wheeler, Rockaway, Garibaldi, and a few other small coastal and dairy communities of Tillamook County. The population of approximately twenty-two thousand, merited a hospital with one hundred beds. The initial survey showed that the district was served by a physician-owned, converted residence-type of hospital and a small maternity home. Together they had about thirty-five beds, none of which were considered acceptable.

In classifying existing hospital beds, designations were made on the basis of whether or not the beds were located in a structure where it would be practical to bring the building up to standards as a hospital or nursing home. The beds in Tillamook County were meeting an emergency need, but they certainly were not "acceptable." I remember my visit to see firsthand the condition of the hospital. It was located in what had formerly been a very attractive, historic house. The interior had large rooms with beautifully grained woodwork, fireplaces, a spiral staircase to the upper floors, and a kitchen and bathrooms characteristic of homes built at the turn of the century. It had been a charming old home but it certainly did not meet the requirements for a hospital. One wondered how seriously ill or injured patients could be carried to the upper floors on that spiral staircase? Obstetrical cases and infants were cared for on the second floor. The only access to the newborn nursery was through the kitchen. The surgery-delivery room and wards were located in what had been bedrooms. It was easy to understand why the staff had classified the beds in this hospital "unacceptable." A maternity home was located a few blocks away in a converted one-story wooden house. Although it had been more recently constructed than the hospital, it too, could not be classified as "acceptable."

The community recognized the dire need for a new modern hospital. It was keenly interested and supported the county court in sponsoring a new facility. Because there were only a few qualified hospital architects in the entire United States at that time, a general architectural firm was employed to draw up plans for the structure. The building was to be multistoried with facilities and the latest type of equipment to care for medical, surgical, and maternity patients. An application for funds and architectural plans were submitted. After a thorough review of the plans, the proposed site for the hospital, the sponsor's qualifications, and the schedule for sound financing, (this was insisted on), the application was approved by the respective authorities.

Funds were allocated, bids were called for, and a contract for construction was let. The hospital was built under supervision of our department and specialized staff of the USPHS. The finest equipment, supplies, and furnishings for all units of the hospital were purchased and installed.

Total cost on completion was approximately one million dollars. This cost of ten thousand dollars per bed for a fully equipped modern hospital was very reasonable compared to costs today.

It was with great pride that the county court, local citizens, officials of the USPHS and members of our Department joined in dedicating this fine new hospital, the first of many in Oregon to be constructed with assistance of Hill-Burton funds.

We have mentioned the fact that the cost of operating and maintaining a hospital over a three year period can equal the cost of constructing and originally equipping the hospital. Too often, sponsors overlook this cost and fail to maintain their fine new hospital. This occurred in Tillamook. Over a period of twenty years, the hospital building was not adequately maintained, nor was it supplied with newer laboratory, diagnostic, and treatment equipment as these were developed. The building had deteriorated. Equipment was old and often obsolete. By 1972, the occupancy rate had fallen to about 40%, although needs for hospitalization had grown. People were leaving Tillamook for hospital care in other areas. With the encouragement of a young physician, Dr. James W. Daskalos, the community was again aroused. County Commissioners leased the hospital to a management foundation. Plans were developed for rehabilitating the hospital. To renovate the hospital a bond issue of $1.6 million was overwhelmingly passed by concerned voters and a federal grant of $750,000 was obtained. The total cost of modernization was almost $2.5 million, (two and one half times the total cost of the original hospital!)

The importance of staying abreast of scientific progress and of maintaining a hospital cannot be over emphasized.

Tillamook united to support one hospital as provided in the State Plan. This proved to be a sound decision. Experience in other areas and studies have confirmed the fact that except in large metropolitan areas, one hospital can be maintained more economically, more efficiently and can provide better service than two or more competing hospitals in a community. Better use can be made of limited professional and technical personnel. Expensive x-ray, surgery, laboratory and other equipment need not be duplicated. Having sufficient beds makes it possible to provide training and experience for interns, residents and other vital health personnel. It is regrettable that in enforcing anti-trust legislation this is not recognized.

State Hospital Plans were based on this principle, recognizing however, that some smaller communities already had more than one hospital. Where these existed, eventual consolidation was sought. Hill-Burton funds were allocated only to those sponsors whose proposals were in accord with the Plan. Some communities duplicated facilities anyway, increasing costs of hospital care in the area. New York state overcame this problem by franchising hospitals. Twelve additional states did this in the early 1980's, in helping to reduce hospital costs. Some of those small communities building multiple hospitals based their decisions on religious differences. Others believed that competition resulted in better service. Another reason given was that an existing hospital did not meet community needs and the administration of that hospital was unwilling to expand or change.

A very complex problem frequently arose when one hospital with a popular staff was overcrowded and applied for funds to expand when the community had a second hospital with many empty beds. Usually, due to community pressure, the more popular hospital was expanded resulting in excess beds in the community. Other complicated problems did arise. The most trying were those involving two applications from a community where planning revealed that a single hospital could best serve the community. A good illustration is that of Salem, Oregon, where two hospitals, Salem General and Salem Memorial, had served the area for many years. Each had made application for funds to build additions or to modernize. Salem General was located on a site with ample room for parking and expansion of its relatively new fireproof building. It had an excellent staff and was well accepted by the community. Salem Memorial also had an excellent staff and was well-utilized. It was located on a relatively small site with limited parking, in an older building adjacent to the Willamette River. Neither hospital was willing to withdraw its application for federal funds.

In an attempt to have the community reach a consensus to support the long-range plan for one hospital in Salem, the community organized a committee of business leaders, professional personnel, and other consumers to study the needs of the area, alternatives for meeting them, and to make recommendations on the provision of additional hospital beds. Ex-Governor Charles Sprague, accepted the chairmanship of the committee. After several weeks of study, further involvement of residents of the area, and with staff assistance in providing requested data, the committee recommended that Salem General be considered as the hospital to be supported for expansion. The value of Salem Memorial was recognized and the committee recommended that limited financial assistance be given to assist it in some rehabilitation, but that it be phased out in future years as more adequate facilities and beds were provided at Salem General Hospital. Based on this recommendation, the Advisory Council on Construction recommended, and the Board allocated, funds to Salem General Hospital for a 60-bed addition in 1953.

The Salem Memorial Hospital Board, medical staff, and community supporters would not accept the findings and recommendations of the local committee. They immediately sponsored a fund drive and built an addition of forty-two beds to their hospital. In 1969, the two facilities merged, eliminating much duplication.

A different situation existed in Pendleton. St. Anthony's Hospital, a Sisters' hospital operated in connection with a church school, was located on a very poor site, locked in by a railroad on one side and a busy transcontinental highway on the other. Only limited parking was available. Expansion could be accomplished with great difficulty and would have to be done largely by expanding vertically. It was recommended that the hospital find a new adequate site considering future needs of the community. Leaders, organizations, and the general citizenry supported this recommendation and agreed to raise funds to help build a new hospital. The sisters however, said that because of the school, they could not move from the existing site. They stood firm. This motivated a community group to sponsor a second hospital on an adequate site. Funds were raised and an application was submitted for a Hill-Burton grant. As this proposal met the standards and requirements of the Hill-Burton Act, a grant was made for the new community hospital.*

These are just a few illustrations of the problem of duplication of hospital facilities. Another problem encountered was that of communities wanting hospitals when they could not afford to build, let alone staff, and maintain them.

Malheur County, Oregon, had an interesting situation with tri-city communities, Ontario, Nyssa, and Vale, located in close proximity. Ontario, the largest, had a hospital, Holy Rosary, which served all three communities to their satisfaction until, 1947 when a polio outbreak was predicted for the area. The local chapter of the National Foundation for Infantile Paralysis

*Disregarding the deficiency in location, as a result of community pressure, St. Anthony's received a grant for a 76-bed addition in 1960.

volunteered to help the Sisters' Hospital develop a special wing for care of polio cases. The Sisters were reluctant to do this. Community leaders made an appeal to district church officials and it was reported, finally to the Pope, but the plan for care of polio patients in the Ontario Hospital was not accepted. Only then did community leaders support a proposal to build a hospital in Nyssa. It was completed in time to care for a number of polio cases.

Shortly after, Vale, the County seat, but still the smallest of the communities with about 1500 population, started a fund drive to build a hospital. The Health Department met with community leaders of Vale and advised that it would not be practical to build a hospital in Vale, not only because of the initial cost, but because of the difficulty in obtaining staff and the cost of operation. A discussion disclosed that the hospital was wanted to attract a physician to the area. The community was advised to build a small nursing home with office and clinic space for a physician and perhaps for a dentist. The facility could be used for emergency care. Some medical and obstetrical cases could be cared for in the home, but it was recommended that the community depend on the hospitals in Ontario and Nyssa, to meet the major hospital needs. This advice was rejected. A fund drive was conducted and sufficient monies were raised to prepare plans, and construct a foundation, outer walls and roof. Funds ran out and the incomplete structure stood empty for many years. Later, it was completed as a community health facility.

The Hill-Burton Act was amended to permit modernization of hospitals and the construction of rehabilitation centers and nursing homes. Although the federal Act provided for diagnostic and treatment centers, only one of these was built in Oregon. It was for out-patient facilities as part of the new teaching hospital at the medical school. A rehabilitation center was added to Emanuel Hospital in Portland in 1961.

The Hill-Burton Act also provided financial assistance in constructing new health department buildings or centers and in equipping them. Several Oregon counties took advantage of this assistance. Many county health departments in these areas were moved from the basements or ground floors of court houses (where most of them has been housed for so many years), to conveniently located and more functional office and clinic space.

As medical science advanced, needs for hospital beds decreased. The original formulas of four and one-half to five and one-half (including beds for chronic disease patients) per thousand population would have provided excessive beds for many states if their populations had remained constant. With rapid growth in Oregon, California, Arizona and other western states the new beds that were provided have been well utilized until recently.* As has been discussed, the Plan was modified each year to reflect population and other changes influencing the need for hospital beds. A marked reduction in the incidence of tuberculosis and need for the hospitalization of psychiatric patients permitted the state hospitals to be used for other purposes.

A few hospitals and a number of nursing homes were built or modernized without federal financial assistance. A beautiful new, hospital, clinic, and teaching complex, Eisenhower Memorial Hospital, in Rancho Mirage, California, was completed entirely with private financial support. Changes in responsibility for Hospital and Related Facility planning began in 1966 when the federal government enacted PL 89-749, establishing Comprehensive Health Planning Agencies both at the state and local level. To illustrate the complications which resulted, in Oregon, a comprehensive Health Planning Agency was established with a State Health Planner.

In 1973, health facility planning was brought under a Health Commission which combined the State Board of Health with the Comprehensive Health Planning Agency. In the same year, the advisory council on Hospital Licensing and two members of the Health Commission were added to a new council. Area-wide Comprehensive Health Planning Bodies were established to cover all of the State of Oregon. Questions arose as to the functions of, and relationship between, the state "Health Commission", and the area-wide Comprehensive Health Planning bodies. Review of Hospital costs by another agency, the Hospital Rate Review Commission established by the Oregon Legislature in 1973, further complicated the relationship of hospitals to government. In 1975, the governor appointed a Task Force to gather information on which Division of the state should implement another new federal Act, the Health Planning and Resources Development Act (PL 93-641). The Governor removed responsibility for health planning from health agencies and assigned it to the Department of Human Resources. In 1977, the Oregon State Health Commission was abolished.

The judgement of professional health people who had volunteered their

*With shortened hospital stays, more surgery being done on an out-patient basis, and with home care many hospitals have an excess of vacant beds and are suffering from financial problems.

services to the state for so many years and the knowledge and experience of qualified health staff having ready access to vital health data and knowledge and experience of hospital and related facility practices was largely lost. Such confusion! It became so great in many states that congress withdrew federal support for hospital planning. Fortunately, sound planning, primarily by State Boards of Health in the early phases of the Hospital Construction and Licensing Programs has been invaluable.

One facet of hospital development that we have not reviewed in much detail is the matter of administration and ownership. We did find that early in the century, the few hospitals that were built were chiefly sponsored by religious organizations, were financed by philanthropists, operated by groups of doctors, or were constructed by government. Most were non-profit. Frequently the administrator was a capable nurse. In mid-century, administration of larger hospitals was in many cases, by physicians or specially trained hospital administrators. Now physicians play a lesser role in administration since non-medical hospital administrators have replaced many of them.

As costs of operating hospitals have risen drastically in recent years, many hospitals have suffered financial losses. Corporations are purchasing and successfully operating chains of hospitals or are contracting to operate "ailing" hospitals. For a time, the government reimbursed hospitals for care on a cost plus basis. There was little motivation for economy, in fact, there was a reward for increasing costs. The government has now changed this policy slowing some of the sky-rocketing costs.

I have outlined experiences in the development of hospitals in Oregon because I was personally involved in much of the early development and was very familiar with it. In general, the experience in the majority of the states was very similar.

Most would agree, in reviewing the record of development of modern hospitals and related facilities, that when Health Departments had responsibility for planning and administration of the construction and licensing programs, they did a commendable job. They were fair, impartial, and free of corruption. The problems in planning and in administration of the programs arose when responsibility was removed from the Health Departments.

11. Preserving Our Teeth: Development of Modern Dental Science

As we consider dental health in this century, we are looking at the creation of a comprehensive service in an important field of medicine. Before discussing health department involvement in the dental health service, it will be helpful to review briefly the development of dentistry as a science.

Prior to 1880, there was a miniscule element of dental practice consisting largely of pulling teeth, filling cavities with lead (in France), tin, or gold, and the making of somewhat cumbersome, carefully carved hardwood, or cast metal dentures. Until 1840, there were no dental schools. The first was established in Baltimore, Maryland, in that year. Prior to that, the occupation was learned through apprenticeship. Abscesses and pyorrhea (infection of the gums), were not recognized or at least not treated. Dental x-rays were not available. Dental caries was a major problem. Occasionally nitrous oxide and ether had been used. Ether was given in 1846 by Dr. William T. G. Morton to extract a tooth, but the use of anaesthetics was relatively rare.

At the beginning of this century, dentistry as we know it today, began to evolve and during the century, developed into an essential art and science.

One of the first major developments was the recognition of the cause and role of tooth decay. Studies to determine the cause were being carried on in Europe. In 1884, Dr. V.P. Miller in Germany demonstrated, for the first time, the role of bacteria, and acid in the process of decay. Thus began an era of change from dental practice consisting largely of extracting natural teeth and replacing them with dentures, to preservation whenever that was possible. Preservation utilized fillings, crowns, (caps), and bridges. Replacement after extraction of natural teeth consisted of providing the patient with partial or complete dentures. With new knowledge, consideration of conditions of the gums, and soft tissue of the mouth, as well as the prevention of dental caries through good dental hygiene, became as important or more important, than structural dentistry. The new concept was embodied in the statement, "with good dental hygiene and dental care, no one should ever lose a tooth."

Surgical and structural elements of dentistry had developed dramatically during the early part of this century. S. C. Barnum initiated the use of a rubber dam around the base of the tooth to be filled or crowned. This rather simple technique was a real boon to success in preventing infection of a cavity being filled, or of a tooth being capped. This practice together with the development of better filling materials such as silver, amalgam, porcelain, cement and porcelain-cement, the use of local anesthetics such as novocaine for less extensive procedures instead of the more hazardous "laughing gas" (nitrous oxide), the use of dental x-rays, beginning about 1910, to aid in finding small cavities, apical abscesses or root involvement and the introduction of dental pulp replacement with gutta-percha or similar impervious material, all constituted major advances in structural dentistry. The use of vulcanized base materials, as substitutes for wood, and cast-metal for partial and complete dentures, constituted further major progress. Extraction of teeth became a refined and skilled procedure replacing rather crude earlier practices. Straightening of teeth was recognized as possible and became more popular as the value of this corrective technique was demonstrated. Orthodontia began to emerge as a speciality in dentistry.

A friend of mine recently told me how her dentist attempted to straighten her teeth when she was about fifteen years old, in the early 1920's. He carefully wired the teeth but unfortunately, his efforts failed. My friend said that she was probably the only patient whose teeth that particular dentist had tried to straighten. Ideas of this kind however, led to better techniques that finally resulted in today's orthodontics.

The most beneficial advances in dental health occurred as recognition of the value of prevention evolved. With the knowledge that bacteria and acid led to tooth decay, studies were made to determine the relationship of dental health to general physical and mental health. Such studies of school children were conducted in Cleveland, Ohio, and Bridgeport, Connecticut, between 1910, and 1919. these studies showed that sixty percent of the children did not use a toothbrush. Many children did not have one! Ten percent of the children had abscesses of their teeth. The author reporting on these studies concluded that in children maintaining good oral hygiene, there was considerably less communicable disease than in those who did not care for their teeth. We now recognize that other factors were involved as well. Another study in Atlanta, Georgia, about the same time, showed that children who brushed their teeth after meals and maintained better oral hygiene, had better attendance records, showed more progress in school, and experienced better weight gain that those who did not.

During World War I, the military for the first time recognized the importance of good dental health and that dental problems could interfere with military activities. As a result, dental units were established to help maintain good dental health in servicemen.

Schools throughout the country began to conduct programs to teach children the importance of brushing teeth and how to attain good dental health. Toothbrush drills were conducted in many schools. Some difference of opinion existed on the best way to brush the teeth. Was a hard, medium, or soft bristle brush or and electric or battery-powered toothbrush best? What should be the shape of and size of the brush? Should a rotary, vertical, or horizontal brushing be practiced? The primary message of the importance of keeping teeth clean however, did make an impact. Later, the importance of flossing, or cleaning between teeth was stressed. Slogans such as "Floss only the teeth you wish to save," and "See your dentist twice a year," were effective.

Another problem that contributed to unnecessary loss of teeth was absence of knowledge or false impressions that parents had about teeth. Not only did many fail to recognize the need for brushing, but many thought that the decay of baby teeth should be of no concern, since they would be lost anyhow. They did not realize that decay of baby teeth could involve permanent teeth. Only the latter were considered to be important. Another misunderstood fact was that six year molars were permanent teeth. Many mothers believed these to be baby teeth and permitted caries* to progress until aching occurred, at which time the teeth were either lost or required capping. I know of persons who had their teeth crowned at that time and have had gold crowns on these teeth for over sixty years.

To illustrate the extent of caries resulting from years of neglect, in examining school children in the thirties, I was appalled at the amount of dental disease which we found in the children in schools. Through

*The decay of teeth resulting in cavities.

cooperation of local dentists in Wasco County, Oregon, and with assistance of Dr. Floyd DeCamp, then Director of Oral Health of the Oregon State Board of Health, dental inspections of over 1300 school children were made in 1938. Only 122 of these children, less than ten percent, did not require dental care. About 400 needed extractions. Over 800 required fillings. There were 460 children who had fillings. About 300 had malocclusions, or faulty closure of upper and lower teeth. While conducting physical examinations of high school children in the Dalles, Oregon, in the late thirties, I found that ten percent of these students had partial or complete dentures! Such findings were not peculiar to this area. In Portland, Oregon, the water supply from the Bull Run River is almost as soft as distilled water. It is used regularly in car batteries. Here dental caries in school children were even more prevalent.

With dental health education in schools, with dental inspections by dentists, physicians, teachers, and school nurses, and in later years by dental hygienists, and with parental cooperation in obtaining dental care for their children, either in private dental offices or in public clinics, considerable improvement was made.

The total dental problem however, was overwhelming. As one dental friend remarked at that time, "There aren't enough dentists to take care of half of the population that needs fillings, extractions, capping, straightening, or other dental care."

Establishment of new dental schools resulted in the training of more dentists, dental assistants, dental laboratory technicians, and later, dental hygienists. This did help.

Another major breakthrough occurred in advancing prevention. It was the discovery of fluoride as an essential element in the formation and preservation of healthy teeth. In the early nineteen hundreds in Colorado Springs, Colorado, Dr. Frederick McKay, noted a considerable difference in the condition of his patients' teeth. Some had a brown stain but otherwise excellent teeth with only occasional cavities. Other patients had no stain but relatively poor teeth with more caries, although they reported brushing and caring for their teeth to the same extent as those with good teeth.

Dr. McKay's practice was unique in that he had patients both from Colorado Springs, which had fluoride occurring naturally in its water supply, and from Boulder, Colorado, whose water supply was without fluoride. Dr. McKay soon correlated the differences with the separate localities, but what accounted for the difference? He made many investigations in the two cities. After several years, he concluded that the difference had to be due to the fluoride content of the water. Colorado Springs residents had the benefit of fluoride in their water, although it was excessive. Those who grew up and lived in Boulder did not. This observation was to benefit millions of children and adults. The problem was how to retain the benefits without the brown stains. State and federal health departments became interested.

Dr. Trenley Dean and a team of USPHS scientists had been studying fluorosis, mottling of the teeth due to excessive amounts of fluoride in water, beginning in 1931. Taking Dr. McKay's observations into consideration, it was determined that one part per million of fluoride in water would greatly reduce caries without causing brown stain. Based on these findings, four-year studies were initiated in New York and Michigan.

An interesting occurrence in Grand Rapids, Michigan, illustrates how emotion can replace sound thinking. Fluoridation was scheduled to begin in early 1945, in Grand Rapids. Unfortunately, delivery of the equipment was delayed by twenty-five days. Shortly after the scheduled starting date, people began to complain of skin rashes, weight gain, and other problems "due to fluoridation." The delay in the arrival of equipment was then publicized. No further complaints were heard! Dental surveys of school children before and after fluoridation and comparison with surveys of school children in neighboring areas without fluoridation showed dramatic differences. In those communities with fluoridated water supplies, the occurrence of dental caries was reduced by over fifty percent, as compared with children in neighboring communities without benefit of fluoride. Extensive studies were made on possible toxic effects of fluoridation at recommended levels. No adverse affects were found.

With the outstanding and overwhelming success of these fluoridation projects—making up a deficiency in water supplies for an essential mineral element that many natural supplies contained—the USPHS endorsed fluoridation in 1951, and recommended that all public water supplies not having naturally occurring fluoride, be fluoridated. After studying results, the American Dental Association, American Medical Association, state and local dental and medical societies, state and local health departments all recommended fluoridation.

One would have thought that with this type of endorsement after the extensive studies, and recognizing the huge problem of dental caries, that every community would institute fluoridation as rapidly as possible. Such was not the case. Legal decisions, making fluoridation subject to public vote, placed it in the realm of politics. Now, contrasting with the experience of chlorination of public water supplies, a segment of the population loudly protested and the question of fluoridation was often put on the ballot. Weird statements were made to the effect that this was a Russian Plot to conquer the United States by "brain damaging the population with fluoride." This was absurd, but I remember that a few prominent physicians in Portland, Oregon, at that time apparently accepted this! One well-known surgeon actually wrote a letter to the editor of the major newspaper opposing fluoridation on the basis of its being a "Russian Plot." Other statements made by opponents of fluoridation were that it was rat poison, it would result in cancer, that it would cause miscarriages, that it would kill goldfish, and that it would ruin gardens and lawns. No scientific data was presented to support their wild claims. It is true that in high concentrations, fluoride can be used as rat poison. It is the dose that makes the difference, as pointed out so clearly by M. Alice Ottoboni, Ph. D., in her book, *The Dose Makes the Poison*. In opponents' claims, no consideration was given to the concentration of fluoride. We have recognized that iodine, chlorine, zinc, and other elements essential to the body's proper functioning, can be toxic if taken in concentrated form or in excessive amounts. Even oxygen, essential to life, can be harmful if given in excessive concentrations. For example, blindness can result form giving too much oxygen to premature babies. In spite of scientific evidence, research support, and the support of recognized health organizations, demands for people to vote on the issue continued. In most areas, voters approved fluoridation and in those communities the incidence of dental caries fell rapidly. More recently it has been shown that fluoride is also beneficial to adults in reducing caries and in helping to reduce osteoporosis or decalcification of bone.

In a few communities, city councils authorized fluoridation as they had previously instituted chlorination, recognizing that this was a public health measure. This occurred in Pendleton, Oregon, in the early fifties. Fluoridation had been carried on for two or three years when a newly-arrived resident, owner of a health food store, upon inquiry learned that the city was adding fluoride to the public water supply. He initiated a campaign to put the matter on the ballot. To clarify the issue, the mayor and council arranged a large public meeting, inviting the protestor, businessmen, physicians, dentists, nurses, teachers, engineers, journalists, reporters, and others who might me interested. I was privileged to attend the meeting. A large group assembled. The mayor explained the purpose of the meeting and then gave the opponent of fluoridation an opportunity to be heard. The protestor was particularly critical of the council for having authorized fluoridation without a vote of the people. When he had finished, the mayor gave one of the finest rebuttals and explanations of the council's action that I have ever heard on the issue. He said that in carrying out its responsibilities to the people, in governing the city, that the council encountered many types of problems. Often these problems were very technical and complex in nature, requiring advice from professionally qualified people. He cited the need for a city engineer because of the many engineering problems, and a city attorney, because of the many legal questions that came to attention of the council. He also mentioned architectural and planning problems requiring consultation from professionals. As the council members were not engineers, attorneys, architects, or planners, they sought the advice of their professional staff or consultants and accepted it.

In this instance, regarding the merits of fluoridation, the council again faced a technical question about which none of the members of the council felt qualified to make a decision. They then called on qualified professional consultants as they were accustomed to doing with such problems. In this case, they turned to the medical and dental professionals for advice. They were then advised by the USPHS, the American Medical Association, and the American Public Health Association that fluoridation of public water supplies as practiced in many communities was a valuable and safe public health procedure. The Oregon State Medical society, the State Dental Association, and the State Board of Health also recommended the procedure. Locally, the Umatilla County Medical Society, Dental Society, and Health Department urged fluoridation. Based on this professional advice, the council, as they had on other technical matters, took the advice of their consultants and authorized fluoridation. It was the consensus of the council that if the members of the council were not qualified to evaluate the evidence and make a decision on such a technical matter, they did not see how the electorate could do so. The mayor had so logically presented the position of the council that there was no rebuttal. The media reported on the meeting, opposition to fluoridation in the city melted away, and the residents of Pendleton continued to receive the benefits of fluoridation without balloting on it.

Fluoridation should not have been a political issue. It is a scientific, medical, and dental health issue which should be decided strictly on its scientific merit.

By the end of the seventies with widespread recognition of the benefits of fluoridation, residents of forty-four of the major cities in the United States that previously had water supplies deficient in fluoride now benefited from it. What a boon to the children in these cities. Chemical analysis revealed on occasion an excess of fluoride in the water occurring naturally in some areas (six parts per million or more.) Growing children drinking such water over a period of years developed mottled teeth, the fluorosis which we referred to in the USPHS studies. Elsinore, California, was an example of a city having excessive fluoride in its water supply. In this instance, the State Health Department required the city to reduce the fluoride content, and until the city could do so, to provide bottled water for drinking purposes.*

Another advance in prevention about this time in the fifties, came with a related discovery that the addition of fluoride to toothpaste could be beneficial in bathing the surfaces of the teeth with much diluted fluoride. Although the American Dental Association previously had not endorsed a commercial product, because of its proven value, it did endorse Crest ™ toothpaste which contained sodium fluoride as an active ingredient. The use of Crest ™ toothpaste became very popular with a clever advertising campaign which portrayed school children who had used Crest ™ coming home after dental check-ups triumphantly calling out, "Look Mom, no cavities!" Later, other dentifrice producers also offered toothpastes or gels with fluoride. Regular use of this type of dentifrice does reduce cavities.

Other developments in recent years included application of protective coatings, particularly to biting surfaces of the teeth, regular cleansing of the teeth, twice a year by a dental hygienist or dentist, improvements in techniques to straighten teeth, use of plastics, and, as in medicine, the use of better local and general anesthetics and antibiotics. Tooth implants became possible to immediately replace broken or lost teeth.

Provision of dental care through state and local government sponsored dental health clinics for children whose parents could not afford to pay

---

*A related study showing the benefits of fluoride was made by Dr. John W. Knutson, Dental Director of the Division of Dental Health, USPHS, and his associates. They demonstrated the value of topical application of a fluoride solution to children's teeth. A program in three Minnesota cities carried on in 1942, was so successful that a national demonstration program was launched in 1950. It too, clearly showed the benefits and the procedure was adopted.

for care, dental health insurance, usually provided through labor contracts, and a country-wide network of modern dental clinics and offices staffed by well-qualified state licensed dental health personnel, have resulted in tremendous improvement in the dental health of children and adults. The dental profession deserves real credit for promoting the preventive dental health services that have been primarily responsible for these advances. In establishing goals the dental profession has maintained as its top priority programs of benefit to the public. State dental societies and the American Dental Association, ADA, have been leaders in promoting these programs.

People appreciate the value of sound teeth and good dental care. This was clearly demonstrated in a program developed in a borough of New York City. A medical clinic was established to care for elderly persons who were known to be without much health care. It was located in an area convenient to most of the elderly in the area. It was modern and well-staffed. Complete physical examinations, x-ray and laboratory exams, nutritional advice and physical therapy were all available. However, very few people took advantage of this health clinic. Perturbed by the lack of acceptance, the sponsors made a survey of the area to find out why the elderly persons did not avail themselves of the service and what they wanted in the way of health care. The results of the survey were revealing. What these folk wanted most was good eye care, dental care, and care of their feet. They wanted to be able to read newspapers and magazines, they wanted useful teeth in order to enjoy their food and they wanted care of their feet so that they could more readily get around. They wanted services of ophthalmologists, optometrists, and dispensing opticians, they wanted dental care, and they desired the services of podiatrists. When the dental, eye and foot services were included the entire clinic became well-utilized. This illustrates the public's recognition of the importance of dental health. Inclusion of dentists on hospital staffs, reflected general acceptance of dentistry as an important arm of the medical team.

We have observed a new health science and profession develop to attack and largely resolve a massive dental problem. Health departments have established dental health programs in cooperation with the dental profession to promote improved dental health. They have sponsored clinics for corrective dentistry for children. They have conducted dental health surveys where needed. They have promoted fluoridation, carried out topical fluoride programs, and have aided in massive dental health education programs. These developments in many areas have resulted in classrooms of children whose smiles reveal well-brushed, well-cared for, sound teeth. This, together with greatly improved adult dental health represents a major step toward better health.

12. Environmental Surveillance for Better Health

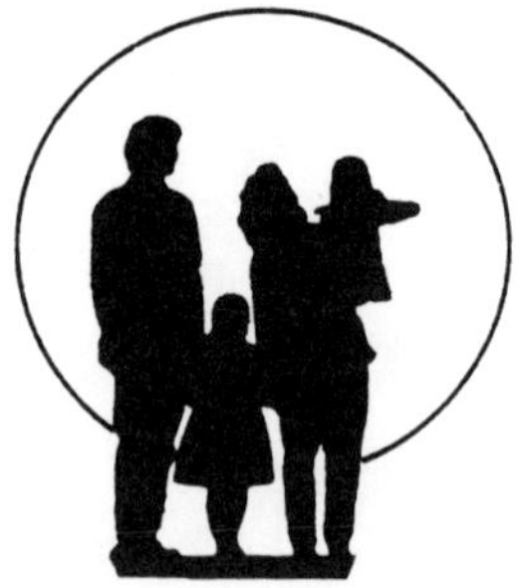

ANOTHER AREA OF major concern to health departments has been the environment. What was the environment like in the early part of the century? The facets are so numerous that it would be confusing to try to discuss them all in chronological order.

WATER

As purity of water became the first serious public health concern in the last half of the nineteenth century, (largely as a result of the recognition of polluted water as the primary source of cholera and typhoid fever), we will discuss water first.

As America developed it was more concerned with an adequate supply of water than it was with purity of water. Cities usually obtained their water supplies from nearby rivers or lakes. In rural areas, many people had springs or dug shallow wells which provided ample water. A few might have heard of poisoned water holes in the west, but water as a source of illness was considered to be rare. Flowing rivers and streams were thought to purify themselves and in any event, how could clear, cold, mountain water contain anything that would cause disease? The occurrence of cholera, typhoid fever, and other dysentery diseases, although suspected by some, were not related to polluted water until the discoveries of Dr. John Budd. in the early 1850's. Snow showed that polluted water accounted for much of the cholera in England, and Budd proved that polluted water supplies were the major sources of typhoid fever. As this knowledge spread, communities became more concerned about their water supplies. They generally had been aware of the practice of cities, towns, or villages upstream, dumping raw sewage into rivers and streams, and coastal cities discharging sewer wastes into ocean bays or into the ocean itself but very few people had any concern about these practices. Now, however, they grew alarmed.

As we have seen, at the turn of the century, cities and states established boards of health to control communicable diseases and with responsibility to assure safe water supplies. Many communities established protected watersheds, (located where they could do so), built dams to impound inland waters, and piped water for many miles to assure an adequate supply of water relatively free from contaminations. State and city health department laboratories checking samples of public water supplies often found E. coli, a bacterial indicator of animal pollution. This data, together with continued occurrence of typhoid fever and other dysentery diseases, led to the requirement and practice of chlorinating public water supplies. Supplies obtained from deep wells were generally excepted as this source of water, filtered underground by nature, was usually pure. Chlorination was authorized by city councils or water boards as a necessity to protect the public health. The resulting reduction in the incidence of typhoid and other dysentery disease was dramatic. It proved the effectiveness of this safeguard.

The CDC made a study of summertime gastrointestinal illness in six Rocky Mountain communities in 1957 and found significant relationships between quality of water supply and illness. Chlorination was recommended.

There was little opposition or fanfare when chlorination was introduced. Occasionally a remonstrance was heard to the effect that chlorine in the water killed goldfish, and rare plants, or ruined lawns. I remember a letter to the editor of an Oregon newspaper, written by a physician-surgeon, claiming that ulcers of the stomach were being caused by chlorination. He apparently had over-looked the fact that the stomach generates a level of hydrochloric acid sufficient to help digest food.

Before leaving the subject of water supply and chlorination it would be well to discuss two related matters. Reference was made to the general belief that underground, or deep well waters were safe and that they did not require chlorination. While the water was usually pure, possible contamination in the distribution system was over-looked. The latter was a potential hazard. An outbreak of typhoid fever in Zurmott, Switzerland, in 1963, was a classical example of a failure in the distribution system due to a contamination of an old water line from an adjacent, equally old, sewer line.

Outbreaks of salmonella in Portland, Oregon, and in the city of Riverside, California, which we reviewed earlier, emphasize this hazard and the need for chlorination of deep well water supplies. Most states have adopted regulations requiring this.

With establishment of county health departments providing supervision of smaller community supplies and with supervision of public carrier supplies such as railroads, airlines, and buses, by the USPHS, water supplies in the United States became among the safest in the world. The USPHS adopted Recommended Standards For Water Supplies. These were adopted by most states. Until recently, as Americans, we have come to take the safety of our public water supplies for granted. It is only when you travel or live in some of the developing countries of the world without such a resource that you fully appreciate how valuable safe water is to us. Our concern now is the possible contamination of water supplies with toxic waste from toxic waste dump sites, chemical plants, service station storage tanks, and other possible sources.

We have considered the hazard of bacteria in water and how this problem has been largely resolved. Recognizing that water could contain minerals and chemical compounds, some possibly injurious to health, chemical analysis of water supplies has been instituted on a regular basis.

One chemical, nitrate, found in occasional water supplies, when ingested by infants, can result in a condition called methemaglobinemia, a form of anemia. As this affects only small infants and occurs rather rarely, residents of areas found to have such a condition are warned of the hazard and advised of how to protect infants in the area.

More recently, concern has been expressed over the finding of asbestos fibers, small amounts of detergent, toxic mineral elements, and minute amounts of pesticides that in rare instances have found their way into the water supply. Pollution of our underground water stores, the aquifers, with toxic materials, became an increasing problem. We will discuss this in more detail later.

With the recognition of the hazard created by communities discharging raw sewage into rivers, bays, and the ocean, governmental action was demanded. Cities downstream from the polluters, growers, and harvesters of shellfish, sportsmen, medical societies, and state and city health departments protested loudly and effectively. As a result, many states enacted Purity of Water laws. Pennsylvania, for example, enacted such an act in 1905. In the early twenties a number of state sanitary water boards were established to function in cooperation with or as a part of a state health department. The USPHS had primary responsibility for water pollution control, at the national level, although the Bureau of Fish and Wildlife, US Corps of Army Engineers, and other federal agencies were also involved.

These agencies initially were concerned with municipal sewage disposal. Treatment of sewage before discharge into rivers, or bays was required. In 1945, 9,000 communities having a population of 75 million people had sewer systems, 5,307 of these had primary treatment plants serving a population of 47 million. By 1962, 11,431 communities with 9,177 treatment plants served 120 million people. Federal and state funds assisted communities in building the treatment plants.

Initially, only primary treatment of sewage discharge was required. Now secondary and even tertiary treatment is often required depending on circumstances. Effluent can be treated to result in water that is sufficiently pure to use it for lakes in parks for recreational purposes.

An interesting problem in control of raw sewage occurred in the mid-forties at a naval base located near Astoria, Oregon. The Navy planned on building a Naval hospital at Astoria, and because it was to be located adjacent to a large tidal basin, proposed to discharge sewage from the hospital directly into the bay without prior treatment. The Oregon State Health Department informed the Navy that treatment of the sewage prior to discharge into the bay would be required. Initially, the Navy refused. They stated they did not have sufficient funds to build a treatment plant. We informed the Commanding Officer of the Base that if they discharged raw sewage into the bay, we would hold the Navy responsible for any occurrences of dysentery disease occurring in the civilian population of the area. We were aware of the fact that many Navy men, exposed to or suffering from Oriental dysentery diseases would be treated at the hospital. The Navy apparently was unwilling to assume the responsibility as a sewage treatment plant was built.

With reduction in municipal sewage pollution, concern over industrial pollution developed. We cannot discuss all of the types, but a sample will give one an idea of their scope. Pollution varied from wastes such as brine from oil refinery operations, coal mine acid waste, sulphite liquor from pulp mills, residue from chemical plants, to biological wastes from logging and lumber mill operations, canning, and poultry meat processing. Potential hazards of thermal and nuclear radiation became evident in the latter part of our century. As standards were established, industry developed new techniques, governmental enforcement spread, and public concern grew, considerable progress was made in reducing this pollution. Industry often found that elimination of waste resulted in financial savings. Oil refining plants that had been dumping brine into small streams, destroying fish and vegetation for miles downstream, were required to stop this practice. As an alternative, brine was pumped into abandoned wells that had been pumped dry of oil. The salt brine, in many instances, brought residual oil to the surface. This oil was recovered, Streams were restored to their natural state.

By 1962, of some 10,500 industries in the United States almost 7500 provided treatment of wastes. To detail the many developments in water pollution control in the various states would require volumes but recounting a few of the experiences which I had will reflect how programs developed throughout the country.

In Oregon, through the efforts of the State Sanitary Authority and the State Board of Health, great progress was made in the late forties and early fifties in cleaning up pollution of rivers, and bays of the ocean, resulting from discharge of sewage from municipalities. One of the major rivers, the Willamette, flowing through a valley in which over a million people resided, was largely freed of sewage pollution. Cities along the river had built treatment plants that were well maintained. The State sanitary Authority, staffed by the Board of Health, was satisfied with the progress of the cities but was concerned with industrial pollution, largely by two pulp mills located on the river at Oregon City. The sulphite liquor waste discharged into the river by these two mills depleted as much oxygen in the river as would a city of 300,00 population. The Sanitary Authority, presided over by Harold Wendel, president of a major department store in Portland, had cited the two mills to hearings year after year because of the pollution. The response of the mills routinely was that means for eliminating the sulphite liquor was unknown but that the industry was researching the matter. In 1955, the two mills, Crown-Zellerbach and the Publisher's Paper, were again cited with the same response. Enough was enough! The Authority told the representatives of the two companies that out of fairness to the residents of cities who had spent millions of dollars to eliminate pollution of the Willamette, pollution by the pulp mills could no longer be tolerated. The mills were given one year to eliminate the pollution or close down.

There was no political interference. It wasn't long before both pulp mills had resolved their pollution problems. Crown-Zellerbach built a large lagoon and stored the sulphite liquor waste in it during the summer months. The waste was pumped out during the winter and spring when dilution in flood water made the waste innocuous. This solution was accepted. Publishers Paper, unfortunately, because of their location on the river bank, could not construct a lagoon of the size required to store the discharged liquor waste during the summer and early fall months. The plant solved this problem by using barges to carry the waste to the Colombia river where the flow was adequate for dilution. As a result of this reduction in industrial pollution, the river was returned to a viable state. The following August, trout were caught in the river at Portland, below the location of the two pulp mills. This proved the success of the control program.*

About this same time, another company proposed to build a pulp mill near the Oregon coast and requested permission to discharge the waste of the mill into a coastal stream. The Sanitary Authority refused to approve the proposal. The Authority required that any waste from the mill that was planned would have to be piped, not to the river's outlet, a bay in which oysters were being grown, but several hundred feet out into the ocean. Officials of the company appealed to the Governor and threatened to build the plant in California if their proposal was not approved.

Soon after the company's threat to build in California, the Governor called and expressed concern over possible loss of the plant. He urged leniency. I explained that the decision was not mine to make, but that I would be glad to present his request to the Sanitary Authority. After considering the Governor's request, the Authority reiterated its position. Mr. Harold Wendel, President of the Authority, called the Governor who again requested approval of the pulp mill's proposal. Mr. Wendel replied that if the Governor insisted on approval for the mill to discharge sulphite liquor waste into the coastal river, rather than pipe it out into the sea, that he and most of the members of the Authority would resign and explain to the media the reason for their resignations. The Governor acquiesced. The company built the plant in Oregon, and met the requirements. Is it possible that actions of State Boards of Health and other non-political agency actions similar to this action led to their demise?

The pollution that we have been discussing has been gross pollution

---

*It is interesting to observe that although the media had noted the success, and the return of trout, a subsequent Governor a few years later, took credit for cleaning up the Willamette River!

with sewage or obvious industrial waste. In the later forties and fifties, health authorities became concerned with less apparent pollution, particularly of ground water, the aquifers, that source of water obtained from deep wells. The USPHS financed studies to determine what hazard might exist from seepage through landfills of refuse and garbage to underground water. With the increased use of very toxic pesticides in agriculture, studies were made not only of the hazard to personnel working with or around the chemicals, but of possible contamination of water and air with the chemicals. Attention was given to asbestos occurring in some water supplies and the possible hazards to health. Safeguards were established to minimize such hazards.

One of the major problems in industry was the disposal of toxic waste. This included acids, and toxic chemicals that had no commercial value, by-products of industrial processes. They were usually concentrated and could not be discharged legally into sewers. Often they were placed in truck tanks or drums and hauled to a site that was considered to be safe for disposal. These sites were carefully selected and had characteristics of what were thought to be large, natural, impervious basins. One of these which I encountered was Stringfellow Quarry toxic waste pit in Riverside, County, California. Toxic wastes from the Los Angeles and adjacent areas had been hauled to and had been discharged there for many years without incident. Illegal roadside dumping was rare. The Riverside County Health Department became concerned with the finding of a trace of chrome compound in well water located at a school some two miles distant from the waste disposal site. This was a new finding and the Department concluded that the only possible source of the compound was the Stringfellow quarry. Although the quantity present was minute and not toxic in that concentration, we feared additional contamination. We immediately recommended to the County Board of Supervisors that application for renewal of a permit to use the site as a toxic waste disposal site be denied.

This recommendation engendered a great deal of discussion. Was there a hazard? Did the contaminant come from the quarry? Where would these wastes be disposed of if this site was closed? Would other means of disposal, some illegal, such as roadside dumping, present a much greater hazard? Parents of school children in the area appeared before the Board, supported the recommendation of the Health Department, and demanded closure of the site. The Board of Supervisors concurred. The application for renewal was denied, and the quarry was closed to further dumping. Cleanup of the site however, presented a major problem, not yet resolved.

An illustration of the hazard of illegal roadside dumping occurred in Riverside County and was brought to light when a flood, actually two floods in early 1969, turned a placid, often dry, river into a torrent. Forty or fifty iron drums, containing a very toxic waste, were exposed when the sand covering them was washed away. Some were rusted and broken. The contents were so hazardous that our Health Department staff and others dared not handle the drums. March Air Force Base came to our aid with trained chemical disposal personnel, special equipment, protective clothing and masks, and removed the hazardous drums. Neither police nor health authorities were able to find the source of the waste which had been dumped and buried many years earlier. Who would ever have suspected that these drums would later be exposed?

In the late sixties, because the USPHS "wasn't moving fast enough", the federal program was reorganized and a newly-created Environmental Protection Agency, EPA, was given the responsibility for water pollution control. Lawyers were appointed to most of the top administrative positions, including the Directors of Regional Offices. Appropriations were increased by congress from the $10.3 million per year level in 1963 for water pollution control subsidies to $1⅓ billion dollars per year in the mid-eighties. This amounted to over one hundred times more than had been spent in 1963! Responsibility for control of expenditures of this amount of money is tremendous. Contrasted with the impartiality and absence of politics in administration of the environmental pollution control programs, by the USPHS, after assignment of responsibility to the EPA, the administration of the EPA was being charged with inefficiency and playing political games with the program. Any increase in effectiveness of pollution control through the EPA came at a huge price.

The EPA was also given responsibility for other environmental pollution problems including air pollution, toxic waste, and clean-up of toxic waste disposal sites. Many of the latter posed major hazards to the health of residents in the area of the sites. Congress established a Superfund of hundreds of millions of dollars to clean up these dumps. According to a series of articles on the environmental "mess", in Newsweek magazine, more than 80% of Superfund spending has gone to consultants and their kinsmen, not to the clean-up of the actual waste dumps.

The EPA was very successful initially in their public relations and relationship with the media. They widely publicized problems and accomplishments. But cost effectiveness has yet to be determined.

MILK

Turning away from environmental pollution, let us reconsider an early public health concern related to milk supplies. Although milk and other dairy products were recognized as important nutrients, they were responsible for some disease in humans. In the early part of this century, tuberculosis of the intestinal tract and bones were related to tuberculosis in dairy cows. Undulant fever was found generally to be the result of drinking milk from dairy cattle or goats infected with Brucelli (abortus or melitensis) respectively.

Early in the twentieth century the federal government, through the U.S. Department of Agriculture, established programs to compensate farmers, first to eradicate tuberculosis in cattle, and then to eradicate brucellosis. By the late twenties, tuberculosis had largely been eradicated in dairy cattle. Tuberculosis of the bone and intestinal tracts in humans became a rarity. Brucellosis continued to be a problem. The Department of Agriculture isolated herds and condemned cows found to be infected. This program and the pasteurization of milk largely eradicated undulant fever.

In many areas, Health Departments inspected dairies and checked on all aspects of milk production and processing. Pasteurization was recommended, but Health Departments insisted that it be properly done. To illustrate, in Wasco County, Oregon, the Health Department found a small dairyman selling what was purported to be pasteurized milk. On testing, the milk was found to be raw. The dairyman did not have a pasteurizing plant. He said that he had been heating the milk in boilers on the stove in his wife's kitchen. Later he did purchase a small pasteurizing plant, but apparently thought that just having one would suffice. Subsequently, the health department revealed that the dairyman had not been operating the plant. The milk that he was selling as pasteurized was still raw. The sanitarian was able to prove this and the Department brought about complete compliance.

Health Departments recommended pasteurization because even with the most sanitary control of milk production, the hazard of a cow developing mastitis, infection of the udder, caused by streptococcal or staphylococcal bacteria, exists. It is not practical to examine the milk from every cow every day and before evidence of mastistis in the cow is discovered, the milk, if not pasteurized, can cause serious illness. Other infections such as Salmonella and even diphtheria have been traced to use of raw milk.

In 1927, the USPHS adopted a Standard Milk Ordinance and Code. These applied to milk shipped between states but many cities and some states adopted the standards. Kentucky, Mississippi, Alabama, and North Carolina were among the first. Dairy inspection and responsibility for maintaining standards initially was the responsibility of state and local health departments. In Oregon, this was true until 1947. The State Department of Agriculture had been responsible for restaurant sanitation. In 1947, the Oregon legislature transferred responsibility for restaurant inspections to the Oregon State Department of Health and responsibility for milk to the Department of Agriculture. The Health Department was given the authority to check on dairies in they were thought to be involved in communicable disease. This exchange of responsibility proved to be of value.

Improvements in dairy farm sanitation, health of dairy cows, refrigeration and transportation of milk, and pasteurization techniques have resulted in a high quality of milk than not only is more palatable, but is also nutritious and safe. Now, milk and other dairy products are processed to keep for days, or in some cases, weeks, and are generally sold in stores or markets. This method of distribution largely replaced the practice of daily home delivery of milk, initially by horse and wagon, and later by dairy trucks.

Another dairy product, cheese, that has become a mainstay in our diets, early in the century was occasionally found to be a source of brucellosis (undulant fever). The source was cheese made from unpasteurized cow's or goat's milk. Ordinarily goat cheese was imported although some was produced in Colorado and other states. A requirement that cheese be produced either from pasteurized milk, or that it be stored for ninety days or more eliminated this hazard. New York state pioneered this requirement.

FOOD

With the attention given to water and milk supplies, assurance of sanitary processing and sale of other foods was initiated. Departments of Agriculture, federal and state, were given responsibility for supervision of meat, poultry and many agricultural products. Nationally the Food and Drug Administration, FDA, was given responsibility for maintaining high standards of food, for processing, canning, and certifying as to the safety and value of drugs. Many states adopted similar laws. California established a Food and Drug Control Program in the State Health Department.

In the early twenties, an episode occurred in California that was to affect the entire canning industry. As discussed in the section on botulism, an outbreak of botulism resulted in a new set of standards for the industry. These served as the basis for national standards. In recent years there has been some problem from customers tampering with foods and drugs. Safeguards in packaging have minimized this.

OTHER HAZARDS

Another environmental problem of major concern in the early part of the century was disease-transmitting insects. The prevalence of Anopheles, Aedes egypti, and other disease-carrying mosquitos, particularly in the southern areas of the country, posed a major public health menace. Malaria, yellow fever, and equine encephalitis were the more common illnesses transmitted by these mosquitos. Initially, control measures involved destruction of mosquito breeding places by draining swamps, oiling ponds, and controlling water levels in canals and other waterways. Education of the public on the value of screening was helpful. Then in the forties, the insecticide, DDT, was discovered and it was widely used to effectively destroy the Anopheles and other mosquitoes in areas with malaria. Mosquitos became DDT-resistant however, requiring the use of other chemicals.

Flies were known to carry typhoid fever organisms and other dysentery bacteria. Through public education programs to reduce breeding places, to screen them out, and to "Swat that fly"; conversion of transportation from animal-drawn to motor vehicles; and better sanitation practices in farm yards; the fly population was reduced. Foods were protected from flies. These programs virtually eliminated flies as an important element in the spread of dysentery diseases.

In some areas where residential development encroached on poultry ranches, dairy farms, and horse ranches, flies could become a real nuisance and threat to health, at least to the emotional well-being of residents in the area. I had occasion to inspect a residential sector in close proximity to a poultry ranch in Riverside County in the early seventies. I could hardly believe what I saw! The walls, windows, doors, and patios of a home were covered with flies, a thick layer — "blankets" of them. Residents could not open their doors without permitting a swarm of flies from entering their homes. I have never seen such a concentration of flies before, even in India. Poultry ranchers cooperated, but it was very difficult to control the fly population. Some ranchers went to the extent of completely encasing their large poultry houses with screens. The ultimate answer had to be to stop new housing developments in the vicinity of poultry ranches or to move the ranches away from residential areas.

Rats, bats, ground squirrels, mice, and roaches were also found to be health hazards. We discussed earlier how plague had occurred in port cities of California. Harbor rats in these cities were the source of fleas carrying bubonic plague responsible for outbreaks early in this century. Fortunately, outbreaks were limited. Plague organisms can be found in ground squirrel populations in western states today, if one looks for the infection. When this happens, baiting programs are initiated, particularly near camp sites and public parks, to kill off the ground squirrels. Educational programs are carried out to warn the public of the hazard of handling sick or dead ground squirrels.

Dogs, bats, and even cats are subject to rabies if bitten by an afflicted animal, usually wild. Many communities require vaccination of all dogs against rabies and recently vaccination of cats also has been recommended.

The small turtles sold as pets for children were found to harbor salmonella organisms. Parakeets could become infected with psittacosis, or parrot fever. Here, again, hazards have been publicized. Restrictions on import, inspection, and transportation of birds subject to psittacosis were imposed by the USPHS and by some states. With uniform federal and state regulations, inspection and certification of the health of birds, cooperation of bird dealers, and education of the public as to the hazard, psittacosis has been controlled.

All of these hazards to health emphasize the importance of Health Department vigilance.

The necessity of surveillance of restaurants became evident in the early part of this century. Initially, responsibility for inspection was often placed, as has been mentioned, with State Departments of Agriculture and, in larger cities, with Health Departments. As occurred in Oregon in the mid-forties, with the realization that Health Departments were better equipped to supervise restaurants, many states delegated the responsibility to establish and maintain standards of restaurants to Health Departments. In the early seventies with the increased interest in environmental protection, responsibility for maintenance of health standards in restaurants was transferred by a few states and counties to environmental protection departments. On first seeing a restaurant license issued and posted by an Environmental protection Department, I couldn't help but wonder whether the interest was in protecting the health of the people or in protecting the environment. Were the personnel in these new agencies as well-oriented to public health aspects and potential for causing illness in a restaurant operation, as Health Department staffs?

The USPHS established standards for restaurants. Most states adopted these or similar standards.* One of the early controversies that arose was between those who believed that a restaurant should either fully meet the standards and be licensed, or license be denied and the restaurant closed. Another group believed in licensing restaurants using a grading process.

Many communities successfully used the technique of grading. A grade of "A" was issued if the restaurant met all requirements. A grade of "B" was issued to those meeting only essential requirements and Grade "C" to those deficient in one or more of the essential elements. The latter was issued for a period of thirty days. If the establishment did not meet the requirements in that time, it was closed. If a deficiency was found that obviously was a hazard to health, for example, inadequate refrigeration of food or unsafe dishwashing practices, the restaurant was immediately closed until the condition was corrected.

Grade signs, particularly the "B" and "C" signs were frequently "lost", or placed in an inconspicuous place by the proprietor. This practice was stopped by the use of decals applied by Health department staff in a prominent place near the entry. Decals gave the grade. The public appreciated this grading program.

Grading gave an incentive to restaurant owners to achieve and retain a Grade "A". The sanitarian, faced with a decision as to whether to close a restaurant if it failed to meet all requirements, and knowing that such closure could deprive the operator of his livelihood, often extended the license, even though he or she was aware that deficiencies existed. In the instance of grading, the Sanitarian lowered the grade until requirements were met. Grading would seem to be the more realistic, the most fair, and the most effective policy.

In many areas, courses of instruction were given to the owners, managers, and food service personnel explaining and demonstrating to them how to serve food without handling it, rather than being "food handlers". The reasons for not handling food were explained. Periodic surveys of all restaurants were made and the results published.

Though the public usually supported and appreciated these measures, it too, needed to be informed on the need for good sanitary practices in restaurants. Early in the Oregon program, in the late forties, we were faced with a situation in a sparsely populated rural eastern Oregon community,

---

*Provisions for adequately washing dishes; refrigeration of foods subject to proliferation of bacteria; protection of foods from contamination from insects and rodents; adequate facilities for cooking and serving food; restrooms; cleanliness of premises; and having personnel trained in serving food safely.

in which the operator refused to comply with the state requirements. She washed dishes in a pan, rinsed them in another, and dried them, too often with soiled towels. Refrigeration was inadequate, and the place was not clean. We recognized that the cafe was meeting a community need, and attempted to help the operator attain a standard of safety. Actually she was operating without a license of any kind. Due to continued hazardous practices, we finally persuaded the District Attorney of the area to issue a legal notice to close the restaurant. The owner consulted an attorney, asked for a jury trial, and the jury found the proprietress "not guilty". Apparently the woman was as unqualified at business as she was in meeting health standards. She voluntarily closed shortly thereafter. This was a rare incident, however. Restaurant operators usually were very cooperative. Owners have discovered that maintaining a high standard of sanitation and cleanliness is just good business.

Plumbing and electrical standards were established early. The objective of plumbing regulations was usually to assure installation by qualified plumbers, use of materials and equipment to protect wholesomeness of the water supply, and the safe disposition of waste. It was also intended to protect against such hazards as explosion of hot water tanks due to uncontrolled heating devices, and contamination of drinking water due to "cross-connections", or "back flow."

Electrical standards, predominantly established and enforced by Building Departments, were developed not only to protect against fires and their toll on human life, but also to prevent electrical shock which in many instances, could be fatal.

Swimming pools and bathing beaches were not overlooked. Not only was the quality of the water taken into account, but the safety of the swimmers was considered.

Motels and hotels usually were required to meet not only fire safety, plumbing, and building standards, but also sanitary standards. Surveillance of hospitals, nursing homes, and related facilities was accelerated, as we have discussed previously, by enactment of the federal Hill-Burton Hospital and Facilities Construction Act.

Occupational Safety became a concern early in this century. Dr. Alice Hamilton, of Harvard, is credited with being one of the first to be concerned with health hazards in industry, particularly in steel mills. She promoted programs of industrial health and safety. State Industrial Accident Commissions and State Departments of Labor were given responsibility for safety precautions. Their purview included not only mines, industrial plants, and transportation facilities, but also elevators and heating plants. Health Departments co-operated with these agencies.

Another area of concern was for the health of workers. Early in this century, attention was directed not only to safety in rapidly expanding industrial operations, but physicians were finding illnesses form occupational hazards. Coal miners black lung disease was one of the first such diseases to attract attention. The hazards of certain toxic chemicals in manufacturing plants, dusts including coal dusts, excess noise, radiation, exposure to lead and petroleum products, pesticides and many others became apparent. The Bureau of Mines and State Industrial Accident Commissions had reduced the accident rate considerably by the fifties, but little had been done about illness. About this time, with federal assistance, many states established Occupational Heath Programs in state health departments. With specially trained physicians, engineers, other health personnel, special equipment, and supporting laboratories, investigations were made of illness suspected of being related to occupation.

Some of the larger and more progressive industries established their own occupational health programs. Many hazards were identified and were reduced or eliminated. In addition to major problems such as coal dust, asbestos, lead, agricultural pesticides, and hazards encountered in the manufacture and use of toxic chemicals, other hazards were found. Use of x-ray in health facilities, and in industry, as well as nuclear radiation frequently posed problems. Some unusual hazards were also identified.

We discussed an outbreak of ornithosis in a turkey processing plant where thousands of birds were infected. The department of Agriculture inspectors were not aware of the infection in the turkeys until after the Health Department began its investigation of human cases — termed "psittacosis."

Fatal accidents involving planes used in agricultural pesticide spraying, were found in some instances to be caused by sudden illness in the pilots due to inhalation of the pesticide.

In the early seventies, congress pre-empted responsibility for Occupational Health and Safety activities by enacting the Occupational Safety and Health Act. OSHA, the enforcing agency adopted many new regulations applicable nationwide. Enforcement of regulations became a major problem. Unfortunately, with this new program much of the benefit of local involvement in enforcement was lost.

We have mentioned radiation in industry. This became a particular problem in the fifties with nuclear energy, industrial and medical use of isotopes and use of isotopes for research particularly in universities and medical schools. Initiated by the State Health Department, Oregon was the first state to establish a state-wide radiation control program. With federal assistance, a small staff including a radiation physicist, (these were hard to find at that time) was established. Guided by an excellent Advisory Committee using the expertise of scientists, including Dr. Arthur F. Scott, of Reed College, the staff surveyed x-ray units in dental offices, medical offices, hospitals, clinics, chiropractic offices, and even fluoroscopic units in shoe stores. Many units were found to be deficient in controlling scatter radiation. Some operators were found who were not sufficiently trained in the potential hazard of excess exposure to x-ray, not only to the patient or customers, but also to themselves.

Surveys of universities, medical and dental schools, and of industries using isotopes and radioactive materials revealed many more users than we had anticipated. Careless disposal of radioactive waste materials into sewers was occasionally found.

Based on these findings, regulations governing use of radiation in the health field were adopted. Through education and cooperation of users, much of the hazard of radiation was reduced. Similar programs were established in many other states.

Excellent progress was made in control of known sources of radiation into the sixties. At that time, nuclear power was being developed as a source of energy. Many atomic energy plants were built or were under construction in the United States. Great public concern arose for fear of accidents at these plants, which could result in irradiation of large areas around the plants.* An accident at one such plant, Three Mile Island, although safely aborted without loss of life, increased this fear. Another problem of concern was the disposal of radioactive waste from nuclear reactor plants. No satisfactory means of disposal of hazardous waste has yet been found. Radiation, then, remains as a possible hazard to health.

AIR POLLUTION

Another potential hazard to health in our environment is air pollution. Concern first was expressed over the black smoke and soot emanating from industrial and domestic use of soft coal with the greatest protests coming

*As occurred at Chernobyl, Russia, in 1986.

from cities such as Pittsburgh, Pennsylvania, that were producing steel. As industry developed, complaints arose around oil refinery sites, cement plants, chemical plants, pulp mills, and other types of industrial plants. Some efforts were made by industry to minimize this pollution but they were not enough. Increase in automobiles and trucks, with their internal combustion engines, began to add to the air pollution problems. Atmospheric conditions, at times, greatly increased the concentration. Inversion layers of air above cities kept polluted air from rising and being dispersed. As a result, concentration of pollutants increased. Sunlight further acted on gaseous elements to from weak formaldehyde which irritated eyes and mucous membranes of the nose and throat. Because of its popularity, Los Angeles, California, was cited as the prime example of this phenomenon. Many other cities experienced similar occurrences. Many of us have heard of the serious episode which occurred in London, England, as a result of air inversion and the burning of soft coal. The sulphur fumes were mildly toxic and as the concentration lasted for several days many deaths occurred, particularly in elderly persons suffering form heart and lung diseases. A similar disaster occurred in Donora, Pennsylvania.

In the early fifties, states became concerned enough to enact legislation creating state-wide Air Pollution Control programs. Again, Oregon pioneered such a program. An Authority was established functioning through the State Board of Health. Its membership paralleled that of the Water Pollution Control Board with professional, technical, and business people serving on the authority. The State Sanitary Engineer and State Health Officer were ex-officio members. Other states established similar Boards and Authorities, usually in connection with Health Departments.

The problems facing these Authorities were more difficult to solve than those of water pollution. A major factor complicating control was the fact that elimination of water pollution in a plant often led to greater air pollution. Installation of air pollution control devices on vehicles to control one pollutant often increased another. Increasing stack heights on industrial plants often decreased local air pollution but increased it in other communities. Another problem in many industries was the huge cost of controlling emissions from plants that were not initially designed to limit emissions.

Recognizing these problems, Authorities established standards which could more readily be met when new plants were built. Experience showed that with public interest and the proper incentive, great improvements could be made by industry. Pittsburgh, Pennsylvania, is an outstanding example of "renovating" a city as steel plants cleaned up their pollution.

Unfortunately, economic concerns occasionally seem more important to a community than clean air. A good example of this occurred in Albany, Oregon. A proposal was made to build a pulp mill a few miles from the center of a small city. Staff of the State Health Department and Authority, met with city officials and the local Chamber of Commerce to warn them of the pollution of the air with sulphite compounds if the plant were built.

At that time the Board of Health had no authority to prevent construction of the plant. The desire of the payroll that would result was greater than concern over air pollution and the city approved the new plant. After it was built, residents of the area protested about the odor. The Air Pollution Control Authority ordered the plant to install equipment to reduce the sulphur emissions. This was done, but at the same time the plant was expanded. Control devices could not completely eliminate the odorous chemicals. Local residents did become accustomed to the stench. However, occupants of trucks and cars traveling Interstate 5, a major highway by the plant, usually were made well aware of the plant and hastened through the two or three miles of the objectionable odor. Other communities near pulp mills had similar problems.

A large aluminum plant located near Portland, Oregon, emanated fluoride fumes in its operation. Nearby vegetation was harmed and it was claimed in the courts that herds of cattle were severely damaged as a result of the plant's operation. Corrective measures were instituted and the pollution problem was resolved.

Motor vehicle pollution was a more difficult problem. As it concerned many areas of the country, control was largely a federal problem although some states, like California, with its millions of cars and trucks, adopted higher standards than those of the federal government.

These were the types of problems that Air Pollution Control Authorities encountered when first established. Considering the limited amount of financial support, real progress was made. Unfortunately, many of the programs were decimated when a wave of re-organization of Health and Social Services swept the country and career and highly skilled professional and technical people were replaced by political appointees, many of whom had little training or experience in the technical programs they were appointed to direct.

Congress had established the EPA. Responsibility for Air Pollution Control was removed from the USPHS. Attorneys were appointed to most of the administrative posts. Although this action had merit in recognizing interstate and regional problems and in providing for more monies than ever had been available for this type of control, it also had its disadvantages.

Many states withdrew all or much of their support of local programs. Not only were funds withdrawn but many states assumed that the federal government had pre-empted the field and that it should assume all responsibility for control. Many well-qualified public health physicians, sanitary engineers, and other health-oriented, technically qualified personnel, left the field due to policy changes.

Initially, the EPA made good progress. Air pollution control standards applicable to automobiles and trucks, helped to reduce pollution from these sources. Emission standards for various industries were likewise effective. Nature did not always cooperate. Mt. St. Helens literally "blew its top", polluting the air with volcanic ash over an are of thousands of square miles. Rains precipitated emissions from industrial plants as acid rains, producing widespread damage particularly in the northeastern USA. Increasing population, more cars and trucks, and industry contributed to the complexity of the air pollution problem. Whether EPA could cope with these problems, whether it could control pollution at a reasonable cost, and whether it could do so without strangling industrial production, transportation and the economy remain to be determined. Some states like California, having areas with greater air pollution problems than others, and not satisfied with EPA progress, established more stringent control programs. Fortunately, there have been no more "Donoras", as occurred in Pennsylvania, but adequate scientific determination of health effects of current levels of pollution have not been made. Too many associated variables such as weather, temperature, and length of exposure have precluded conclusive proof of health effects except on persons with chronic heart and lung disease. The most conclusive evidence of the results of "personal air pollution" is that of inveterate cigarette smokers experiencing increased numbers of deaths from cancer of the lung, heart attacks and emphysema.

SOLID WASTE DISPOSAL

Before leaving environmental health, we should consider solid waste disposal, the magnitude and character of which has become a potentially major health problem. With increased population, industrial development, and desire for convenience and material comfort, our society became one of the most wasteful in man's history. Millions of tons of waste are accumulated each year, and the disposal problem looms larger and larger. Early in this century, dump sites were usually available. Individuals frequently disposed of their own garbage and trash. In large cities "haulers" collected garbage. Industries frequently disposed of their own garbage and waste on adjacent properties or in streams. Garbage dumps were common. Rats, flies, and mosquitos found harborage in these dumps.

As health hazards became known and with the establishment of Health Departments, cities and counties began to establish "sanitary landfills". The day's deposits were supposed to be covered with soil each day. Only with close supervision however, did this occur. Some people, unless required to do so, did not avail themselves of garbage and trash collection service. In the early forties, I actually saw the backyards of houses in re-development areas of large cities, littered two and three feet deep with discarded, rusting food cans, and all manner of trash. It is still occurring in some neighborhoods. With more efficient collection, with mandatory pick-up, most cities solved the collection problem, but with the massive accumulation of waste and as the landfill sites were exhausted, disposal has become a critical problem. New York City, for a time, barged waste out into the ocean and dumped it. This created serious problems, polluting ocean shores and beaches. The practice was stopped. Proposals were made to fill empty railroad cars and dispose of waste in abandoned mines. This was not practical and met objection from the states designated to receive the waste. Some cities required separation of cans, bottles, paper and trash from wet garbage. Re-cycling of the one type and incineration of the latter is being undertaken. Compositing of wet garbage is being tried. In some areas these approaches are meeting with success although the cost of building the necessary plants has been high. Experimental projects to convert old land filss into landscaped parks are being tried.

We are making progress in solving our waste disposal problems. Disposal of toxic and nuclear wastes constitute our major unresolved ones.

In reviewing the many aspects of our environment in which Health Departments have been involved, it is obvious that protection of the public health has been the major objective. Considering the limited amount of funds and authority available to them, it is apparent that Health Departments, with well-qualified professional and technical personnel, free from political interference, did a reasonably good job. Now Health Departments are often fragmented and responsibilities for environmental health are scattered among many federal, state, and multiple local agencies. Directors of many of these do not have the health knowledge or experience to recognize and resolve the complex public health problems related to the environment. Accusations of corruption in the top levels of government agencies are heard. Considering these recent developments, we might ask: "Have the political administrative changes resulted in improved Environmental Health?"

13. Bookkeeping Of Humanity

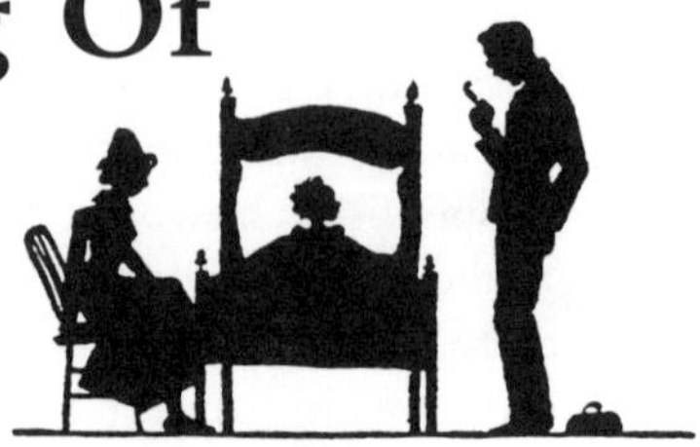

HOW IMPORTANT ARE vital statistics; communicable disease reporting, recording, and analysis; and reporting of various illnesses and evaluation of treatments and progress in combatting them? A review of how our current system developed and of its importance to public health will help us better in evaluating it.

At the beginning of this century there were very few accurate records of births, deaths, other vital events, and communicable diseases. Certainly there was no system of vital records. To create a comprehensive system of accurate records, usually computerized, permitting sound planning and evaluation of the health of the nation and of health programs, has been an impressive accomplishment.

The US Census which was established by Congress in 1790, had been instituted primarily to enumerate numbers of inhabitants in order to determine representation of states in the Congress. As a measure of how far our society has progressed, it is interesting to note that the first Census classed individuals as "free", or "slaves". Age and sex were important as the Census was used for military draft purposes. In 1830, persons who were blind or "deaf and dumb" were recorded as such. There were many inaccuracies and omissions in these early censuses made every ten years. It was said that the 1870 Census was the poorest ever made in the United States. The Superintendent of the Census stated that the federal law providing for the Census was "clumsy, antiquated, and barbaric." There also was considerable controversy as to the role of the federal government and the role of the states, many maintaining that only the states had a right to register births, deaths, marriages, and other vital events.

In 1880, a major improvement was made in the national Census. For the first time, local staff was employed to interview people and to collect data. Because all of the information was not classified, and the vital statistics had to be hand-tabulated, it took almost ten years before complete statistics on the 1880 Census were available.

In 1900, Census data was separated into major and minor classification and in 1902 the Bureau of Census, for the first time, was made a permanent part of the federal government.

The 1990 census, required for this decade, although flawed with some errors, was probably the most complete ever made in the United States.

At the turn of the century, as states established state boards of health, in addition to other responsibilities they were directed to maintain vital records. By 1900, however, only eleven states provided for registration of births and deaths and it was not until 1933 that all of the states were included in the National Registration System. Mortality, birth, stillbirth, and infant mortality statistics were published intermittently beginning in 1867, but it was not until 1940 that continuous annual publications of this data was initiated.

As people began to recognize the need for birth certificates to establish citizenship, to provide proof of age for entry to school, for drivers licenses, for Social Security registration, and for other purposes, with a much greater proportion of births occurring in hospitals, deliveries by physicians, and with legal requirements, recording of births became much more complete. Those who had not had their births registered could arrange for delayed filing. Affidavits from mothers, records in family Bibles, school records, insurance application forms, census and other similar records were used to substantiate details of birth and file either with a county, city, parish, or state. Standardization of birth, death, stillbirth, and other vital records, and checking of these records for completeness and accuracy, usually by Health Departments, insured ever-increasing improvement in the quality of the records and the statistics from them.

To safeguard the information, laws were enacted to provide for confidentiality. Records were maintained locally with copies sent to the state. In the forties and fifties, many states began to mini-film vital records and to protect the records in case of disaster.

Provision was made for safeguarding information on illegitimate births and on adoptions. This proved to be quite a problem when an adopted child, later in life, sought to learn of the natural mother's identity. Many states require court orders to release this kind of information. Health Departments had strict policies on confidentiality of such information. I remember an incident in the forties when I served as State Health Officer of Oregon, when one of our staff, in filing a record on a birth, recognized the mother as a student in one of the local high schools. The staff member lived in the neighborhood of the high school and one evening, in a conversation with a friend, the name of the high school girl came up and a question arose as to why she had dropped out of school. Our staff member, remembering the birth certificate, inadvertently commented, "Oh, she just had a baby!" Word soon got around. The young unmarried mother was truly embarrassed and reported the incident to our Department. After a fair hearing in which the staff member acknowledged that she was aware of the strict policy on confidentiality, and that she had erred, we found it necessary to terminate her employment. This was a drastic action but confidentiality had to be maintained.

Format of birth records was changed over the years with confidential information, for example, on handicaps, provided for on a detachable part of the certificate. The certificate was also used to determine compliance with the requirement for application of silver nitrate solution or other prophylactic, to the eyes of newborns to prevent gonorrheal infection. The information was used not only to determine incidence of defects and compliance with the law but also to plan programs and to assure service for handicapped persons.

In the sixties, some states prohibited the inclusion of color or race on the certificates. Later, they were at a loss to provide data on racial differences in infant and maternal mortality or incidence of handicaps because they did not have the information.

We had an excellent Bureau of Vital Statistics in Oregon. Deane Huxtable, an able Director of the Bureau for many years, was succeeded by Marian Martin. Both were very progressive. Deane helped convert hand tabulation of records to machine tabulation using punch cards and sorters. Actually, it took fewer clerks to tabulate much more data and probably with considerably greater accuracy than with hand tabulation. Special studies could be made such as on the incidence of handicaps for example. Now computers are used. Annual State Vital Statistical reports were prepared and distributed. These were helpful to many agencies including universities, colleges and schools, hospital planning bureaus of health departments, various voluntary and governmental agencies, and of course to the various program directors of state and local health departments.

The National Office of Vital Statistics held annual conferences of State

Directors of Vital Statistics to get suggestions on needs for changes in standards and procedures, to inform the directors of proposed policy changes, and to improve communication. I remember Deane Huxtable's having suggested an improved numbering system for birth certificates. To me it seemed very logical. Each state would be given a number. Another number would designate the county, and another the city, thus, locating the place of birth. The year, month, and date of birth would also be designated by numbers. Where multiple births occurred on the same day in the same place, each infant would be given an additional number.

This identifying set of numbers could then be used as the Social Security number. It would be much more meaningful and would prevent many abuses of use of Social Security cards. Unfortunately, with memories of the Fascist State of Hitler's Germany, the proposal was rejected on the basis that it would lead to a "Police State", in this country. Would it have been any different in this regard to an assigned Social Security number? Deane gave up the idea and devoted his talents to improving other facets of the program.

Death records were important to families in collecting insurance. Data from them was also very valuable to physicians, to public health departments, medical schools, medical societies, voluntary health agencies, agencies of government, and to researchers. Causes of death were essential to determine frequencies of fatal events, to help establish priorities for programs to prevent various kinds of death, and to measure progress in these programs.*

Death certificates particularly, must be complete and accurate to be of any value. Health Departments helped ensure such accuracy. Local registrars, usually in health Departments, reviewed certificates for completeness and correlation of the stated cause of death with standard classification and nomenclature. Often checks had to be made with physicians to clarify causes of death. Burial permits could not be issued until the certificates were complete. This latter provision helped secure more rapid completion of death certificates.

In most states, when a deceased person has not had a physician in attendance in recent years, or when a physician did not have sufficient information to state the cause of death or complete the death certificate, or

*Again, development of statistics evolved from hand tabulation to machine sorting and now to the use of computers.

when violence was suspected, the case was referred to a coroner. In many areas the coroner was an elected officer of local government. Funeral directors usually held these offices. On receiving reports, the coroner often transported the deceased immediately to his own funeral home. The conduct of the funeral in that home usually was thus assured. When a case was reported from a distant area or one geographically difficult to reach, the coroner often made a brief inquiry, questioned the police if they were involved, and concluded from this information what he or she thought the cause of death was.

Autopsies were ordered in some instances but these did not always detect deaths resulting from crime. Failure to request an autopsy could be a serious oversight. Some states recognized the inadequacy of the coroner system and the need for skilled examiners with training, not only as physicians and pathologists, but in addition, with training in forensic pathology to investigate deaths when cause was questionable. Virginia was one of the first states to adopt a law establishing a medical examiner system.

Recognizing some of the problems with the coroner system in Oregon in the mid-fifties, Mr. Huxtable and I visited Virginia to study the medical examiner system in that state. We were likewise impressed with the skill, techniques, and special knowledge of the forensic pathologist. It was obvious that his or her special training and expertise was invaluable in detecting evidence of criminality or death warranting special criminal investigation. As a result of our study we recommended to the Oregon State Legislature the adoption of a medical examiner system. This required a change in the State Constitution. To convince the Legislature of the great need for this major change, we presented many instances illustrating the inadequacy of the coroner system. One impressive case occurred in Salem, the state capital city. Two men, obviously under the influence of alcohol, checked into a motel about midnight. The next morning a maid, coming in to make up the room, found both men dead. The coroner was called. He made inquiries, learned of the alcoholic state of the men and certified the cause of death of both men as "acute alcoholism." When these death certificates reached the desk of of Dr. Willard Stone, Marion County Health Officer, he questioned the cause of death as given, knowing that under the circumstances, death from "acute alcoholism", particularly in both instances was very unlikely. He and his staff made an investigation, found an improperly vented gas heater, and on further checks of the deceased, found that they had died of acute carbon monoxide poisoning. (What a difference to the families, not only in collecting insurance, but also in their emotional state.) This, and similar case presentations overcame the opposition. In 1959, the citizens of Oregon changed the Constitution to provide for a medical examiner system.

The system was established. Local health officers were designated as local agents of the medical examiner. They worked with police officers. In all questionable cases, the state medical examiner was called in. The system proved to be a major advance in improving accuracy of causes of death where questionable. More recently, many states and major cities have established such systems.

Certificates of marriage and divorce were usually processed by county clerk's offices, but copies of the certificates were transmitted to State Health Departments. This information was analyzed, tabulated, and the results were included with other vital statistics data. Reports on communicable diseases were sent by physicians to the local health officer. Certain quarantinable diseases, or where these were suspected by a physician, were reportable by telephone. Other communicable diseases designated by the state, were reported on a weekly basis. Threatened outbreaks could be anticipated and appropriate measures taken, warning physicians and the public. Local health officers used these reports as a basis for investigations and control measures. Tabulations, annual or more frequently, permitted evaluation of progress in controlling disease.

In certain instances, more detailed registers were maintained in particular departments to assure adequate treatment and follow-up. Such a register was maintained in Oregon for tuberculosis control. A full-time clerk maintained a statewide register using color-coded cards. Local health departments sent in data on each patient, diagnosis, stage of the disease, presence or absence of tubercle bacilli in the sputum, the patient's location in a hospital, sanitarium, or home, and the recommended follow-up by public health nurses. One of the aspects of control was related to reports on patient follow-up. If these were not received, reminders were sent out, requesting information on the results of the follow-up. The register was invaluable at that time. In a matter of hours, or less, the total number of patients with tuberculosis; hospitalized; with positive sputum; and status of follow-up by public health nurses could be determined. Success of treatment, and progress in control was measured. Now, this can all be done utilizing computers.

California maintained a very valuable and nationally recognized Tumor

Registry. Through the cooperation of hospitals and physicians of the state, reports on patients with cancer were sent to the state health department. Diagnosis, type of treatment, and results of various kinds of treatment were reported. Summary data was available to physicians. On request, information on the results of various kinds of treatment was given to the physician. This material was published periodically and was very useful in determining which type of treatment was most successful.

Special studies and reports were made by health departments in various areas of the country on automobile accidents, accidents in the home, various handicapping conditions in children, personal health practices and their effects on longevity, and related subjects.

More could be written on the Bookkeeping of Health, and how it evolved. I have limited our considerations primarily to outlining developments of vital statistics; communicable disease, and other public health records; and in the methodology of collecting them. From them emerge an image of the public's health as portrayed in these accounting books, indeed, the Bookkeeping of Humanity.★

★In some communities, responsibility for maintaining vital, communicable disease and other health records essential to recognition of community health problems and planning programs to protect the public health, has been given to public agencies other than health departments. Often events are merely recorded, and in many instances, seldom, if ever, used to determine health needs, to plan and to evaluate public health programs. Many states are still without Medical Examiner Systems to determine accurately the cause of death.

Evaluation should be made to ascertain how best to collect and utilize such vital information.

14. Promoting Better Health

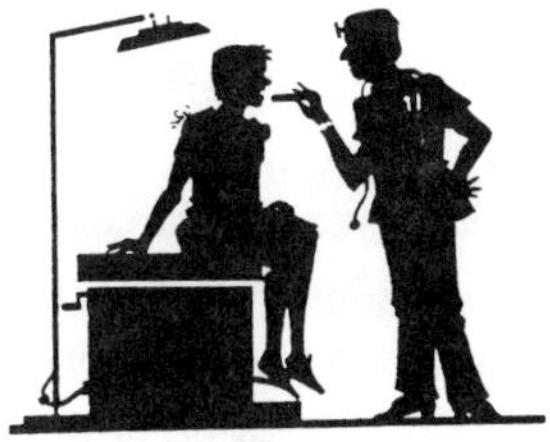

EARLY IN THE century there was very little in the way of organized Public Health Education for the general public. Schools, physicians, and other health personnel provided health information, but people generally learned what little they knew about improving their health from their families and friends. Patent medicine peddlers undoubtedly gave out more misinformation than accurate health information.

With the establishment of state boards of health and with more knowledge on the cause of disease, particularly communicable diseases, the need to inform the public of measures they could take to protect their health soon was recognized. Through the newspapers and magazines of the day, people were advised of the importance of drinking pure water. They were told to boil water prior to using it if it was of questionable purity. Knowing that typhoid fever was spread by the "Four F's: Fingers, Food, Flies, and Fecal material", information was given on how to protect oneself from contracting the disease. Some states had "Swat That Fly" programs. Emphasis was given to screening against flies, and construction of outhouses, or privies to prevent access by flies. Use of sticky flypaper was encouraged. I remember seeing narrow strips of it hanging from kitchen and dining room ceilings. People were urged to wash their hands thoroughly before eating and after toilet use.

Publicizing outbreaks of cases of smallpox and the availability of vaccination motivated many to obtain this protection. With decreases in typhoid and smallpox, attention was turned to other diseases. With the organization of volunteer health agencies, health education campaigns were organized. One of the first was the campaign against tuberculosis. Christmas Seals drew attention to the problem. "Use A Spitoon", "Cover That Cough", and other similar slogans were being used effectively. Old wives' tales were being replaced, in the minds of people, with factual health information.

It would take many volumes to detail the developments in Health Education during this century, but we can highlight some of the major developments. As we discuss programs let us consider Health Education as the more formal type of presentation on health as given in schools and colleges.

Health information would include more informal means of communicating facts on health to the general public. Initially, this type of information was given through newspapers, magazines, public meetings, posters, pamphlets and leaflets, and through the personal contacts of physicians, dentists, nurses, pharmacists, and other professional health personnel, with patients or with the general public.

Education on health in schools in the early nineteen hundreds was gradually incorporated into science and physical education classes. Many states enacted laws prescribing essentials of health that should be taught. Diet, care of the body, toothbrushing, exercise and sleep, and the hazards of drugs, alcohol, and smoking were some of the subjects covered.

Not only was the curriculum changed considerably in ensuing years, to include information on health, but as the science of medicine developed, Health Education became more comprehensive. In elementary schools, responsibility for teaching of health was given to the classroom teacher, In high schools, the physical education instructor was often responsible. Undoubtedly, much was accomplished in the earlier years but questions arose as to the effectiveness of the teaching in actually changing students' health habits. I am reminded of an incident in a rural school in the later thirties in a county where I served as Health Officer.

A Public Health Nurse and I arrived at the school to perform physical examinations. It was just a little before noon. As we entered the one-room school, the teacher greeted us and asked if we would mind if she completed her presentation on Health. Gaining our consent, she went ahead and did an excellent job in explaining how, among other things, disease-causing germs on the hands could enter the mouth in eating and emphasized the importance of washing the hands before meals. Upon concluding the lesson on Health she said, "Now children, it is time for lunch. Take out your lunches and eat. Please hurry, so that we won't keep the doctor and nurse waiting." No provision was made for handwashing, nor was it suggested. This could have been an isolated incident. In this school, water had to be carried into the building in a bucket from a nearby well. This type of didactic Health teaching did not always result in desired health practices. School administrators and health officials recognized this.

In the fifties, the Kellogg Foundation sponsored a number of special projects in some of the schools throughout the country to explore more effective ways of teaching Health. The State Health and Education Departments in Oregon joined in applying for a grant. After the grant was approved, an interested teacher was selected and given additional training in health education. She served as a consultant to teachers in one community. An initial survey in the schools showed that health was the least-liked (actually dis-liked) subject, by both teachers and students. In this project, a new technique, with flexible format, replaced didactic teaching. Consideration and discussion of ongoing health activities was the basis of this teaching. If a case of polio, tuberculosis, or other disease occurred, if there was an outbreak of flu, if an accident happened, or a program of immunizations or school examinations was conducted in the school or community, they were studied in depth. The pupils gathered as much information as possible on the incidents. Discussion included causes, results, and means of prevention when applicable. Students visited the local hospital, offices of doctors and dentists and the health department. They made visits; with the sanitarians to see water supplies, dairies, restaurants, and public swimming pools; and to learn of the work of the health department clinics.

After a year, an evaluation was made of this new technique used in teaching health. Now the students and teachers rated health as their most interesting subject. Not only had students knowledge of health and health practices improved, but some students became interested in health careers. Unfortunately, the special project ended after two years. "Limitation of budget" was given as the reason for not extending the program to other schools. It probably was more expensive and time consuming but it "paid dividends." Certainly the lesson learned on methodology should have influenced the teaching of health in these and other schools.

Later in this century, in the fifties, sixties and seventies with even more scientific knowledge, with more students smoking cigarettes and marijuana, abusing drugs and alcohol and with the change in attitudes toward sex, more effective means of communicating with, or "getting through" to students were needed and tried.

Use of peers, e.g., high school seniors as consultants to freshmen on health matters was one such approach. A successful program of this type was developed in Philadelphia, Pennsylvania. It was aimed at cigarette smoking and drug abuse. In providing family life education, parents were involved in the development of the programs. (In some areas, uninformed parents denied their children the benefit of such education and opposed education on sex for all children.) Many exclaimed that providing such information was the responsibility of the home and the church. However, when queried, very few parents had done so. I have often wondered why such successful techniques are not incorporated into more school programs.

Now, school staff and public health nurses make more use of consultation from Health Educators. Beginning in the forties, Schools of Public Health established courses for Health Educators and trained many. Gradually, they were recognized as essential members of the health team.

The scope and techniques of public health information also changed considerably during this century. Health departments and voluntary agencies took increasing interest in providing the public more health information.*

Business and industrial leaders became interested and provided leadership in promoting better health of their employees and the public. They served as officers and members of Boards, or Directors of voluntary health agencies. They made major contributions to health information programs.

I remember one outstanding contribution in Portland, Oregon, which occurred during the war years of the forties. Aaron Frank was president and manager of a large, central downtown department store, Meier and Frank, the major department store in Portland at that time. Like most department stores, this one had continuous show windows facing the sidewalk and street on all four sides of the building which covered an entire block. In preparation for a regional meeting of the American Public Health Association in Portland, State Health Department staff asked Mr. Frank if we might utilize some of the windows for health displays during the week of the meeting. Aaron Frank was enthusiastic about the prospect. He had a particular interest in helping crippled children. He told us that not only could we have all of the display windows for the week, but he offered the use of the store's spacious auditorium located on one of the top floors of the building. We were quick to accept, and with cooperation of a number of voluntary health agencies, we used all of the display

*Voluntary health agencies increased in number spectacularly with an agency supporting attacks on each of many of our known diseases, abnormalities, and hazards. I was amazed recently in visiting a Medical School Library, to find two large volumes, about 2,000 pages in each, listing, and briefly explaining these and other agencies!

windows—there must have been at least forty of fifty of them—and the health meetings were held in the auditorium that week. Developing that number of good health exhibits and displays was a huge undertaking, but with cooperation of the volunteer health agencies, it was accomplished. The program was a huge success. This, in part, was the result of full-page advertisements in the daily newspaper, arranged by Aaron Frank, featuring the health exhibits and Health Fair. These ads replaced the usual merchandise advertising. The local newspapers and radio stations cooperated in publicizing the meetings featuring health articles and reporting on health topics covered by key speakers. This was an effective means of providing health information.

Health science writers have developed into an important group in researching and writing on health subjects and development. These articles usually are very valuable. Occasionally the media publicizes a development before its merits are proven. This can lead to unwarranted hopes for cure.

Other types of activities to further health programs and to spread valuable health information were inaugurated. The American Medical Association and State Medical Societies had conferences on school health, rural health, industrial health, and similar subjects. In Oregon and other states, teams of outstanding physicians and dentists traveled to many centers throughout the state to present the latest developments in medicine and dentistry to local doctors and dentists, and on occasion, to the general public.

Medical society auxiliaries, health departments and voluntary health agencies often sponsored Health Fairs. Now hospitals are employing Health Educators and likewise sponsor Health Fairs.

Inclusion of Health Educators on staffs of many health departments in state and large city departments of education, in voluntary health agencies, in hospitals and some of larger industries reflects recognition of the need for more health information and has increased its effectiveness. Schools of Public Health not only prepare these professionals in techniques of health education and information, but also prepare them to help organize communities in implementing specific health programs. In the chapter on Tuberculosis Control, I outlined the outstanding community organization feat directed by Mary Jo Kraft, who at that time, was with the Tuberculosis Control Unit of the USPHS. Unfortunately, many health departments have failed to utilize all of the abilities of Health Educators. Emphasis has been given to writing news releases and health bulletins, maintaining health department libraries of books, films, and slides, and developing health literature. The talent for community organization has too often been overlooked. Voluntary health agencies, often directed by persons skilled in health education, recognized the great benefits of mobilizing capable volunteers. They arranged for them to make talks, show films, distribute literature, staff exhibits of Health Shows and Fairs. They recognized too, that people really learn when they are personally involved in health information activities.

Another development has been the establishment of "hotlines." These are telephone answering services that anyone with access to a telephone can contact to obtain health information. Many local medical societies, Riverside, and San Bernardino County California Societies were two of the first to sponsor a telephone center, have tapes on various health subjects. A caller could dial for information on most of the diseases, on nutrition, immunizations, and other health subjects, and would then hear an excellent, brief presentation on the subject. Hotlines were also established to help those with emergency health problems such as drug problems, thoughts of suicide, and complications of AIDS.

Improved techniques including the use of videotapes, closed circuit television, cassettes, computer programs, games and clever visual aids such as cartoon presentation for children, all contribute to more effective education of the public on health matters. Public information given through the media, has grown in importance and has a great influence on health practices. Publicity on "cholesterol" and its relationship to heart disease and high blood pressure, information on HIV and AIDS, and explaining the hazards of cigarette smoking are good illustrations. Head-lining deaths of prominent sports heroes, actors and actresses dying from cancer attributed to the smoking of cigarettes, sway many. Commercial advertising frequently capitalizes on the public's interest in health.

Commentators on health, usually physicians, and TV, radio, and other personalities, generally discussing or answering questions about disease or other aspects of health, have a great impact on the public and generally make a real contribution to better health. Newspaper and magazine columnists likewise contribute.

The Health Departments role in these programs has largely been one of promotion, co-operation, and often in providing accurate information. Their most important role is in providing information on an informal basis in offices and homes. Counselling is on an "eye-to-eye" basis, one of the most effective means of communicating health information to individuals.

Certainly a better informed public has been a major factor in control of many diseases, in better nutrition, and in achieving better dental, physical, and mental health.

A major problem still exists in getting the public as a whole to improve their health practices. To illustrate the problem, education and information on the value of the use of seat belts in cars, and even laws requiring there use, have not been entirely effective. Statements like that of a state police officer with twenty-five years of service that he had "helped pick up many automobile accident victims thrown from a car, but had never found it necessary to unbuckle a casualty restrained by a seatbelt", impress people, but do not motivate them to always use belts. "It will never happen to me", is too common a misconception.

Similar examples could be given on the tragic results of postponing consultation with a physician on early signs of cancer until too late, or failure to follow a physician's or dentist's advice. Abuse of drugs; continued smoking of cigarettes; "burning the candle at both ends", or excessive work, worry and strain; inadequate diet, insufficient sleep, and exercise; are additional examples or poor health practices which we should and must do a better job in changing. Individuals can do a great deal more for themselves in maintaining good health. Health education and providing effective health information are our major tools to help them.

15. Public Health Nursing

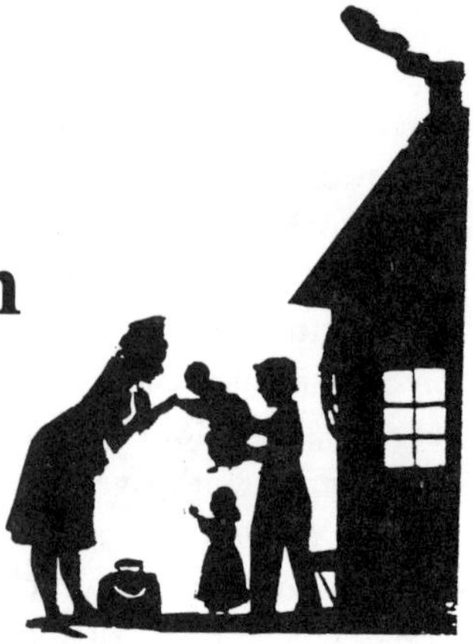

THE PUBLIC HEALTH nurse is an essential member of the public health team. She (or he) is one of the most valuable participants. (For convenience I will use "PHN" or "she" in the designation of the public Health nurse.) One of the PHN's major contributions is the unique value of her visits to the home. Here the PHN provides service in follow-up, in explaining health needs and recommendations of physicians, in individual and family counseling, and in referring those she serves to appropriate facilities for care. If her schedule permits, she is able to develop a rapport with a family or an individual, a personal relationship and acceptance as a friend, which makes her one of the most effective of public health workers in providing information and advice. She is often able to motivate individuals and to obtain essential and valuable information when other measures to obtain it have failed. She can be an extension to the home from the office of the family-practice physician, or other specialist. When given the opportunity and the necessary time she can locate the pregnant women in need of care and arrange for it. She can locate children in need of immunizations and motivate their parents or guardian to obtain them. She can counsel and help others in need of medical care. Too often the value of her service is not considered or is over-looked when plans are made for huge programs such as those to control the spread of HIV infections (ARC and AIDS). Some of us may not be acquainted with the activities of a Public Health Nurse. Many illustrations could be given of the great value of these specialized nurses. Several instance come to mind.

The Chief of the Department of Ophthalmology in a medical school became concerned about the number of patients who failed to return for check-up after eye surgery and who lost more sight. Public Health Nurses who were called in to assist, visited patients in their homes and learned, in many cases, that the patient's expectations for improved sight had not occurred. They became disappointed and often failed to use prescribed drops, to follow doctor's orders, or to return to the clinic. The PHN was able to explain in detail that in many cases the surgery was intended to retain vision and to prevent further loss of vision. She was able to answer questions to reassure the patient and to persuade him or her to see the ophthalmologist again. This service proved to be invaluable and undoubtedly helped to save the sight of many.

Earlier I referred to the completeness of public health services in the Wasco-Sherman Counties, Oregon, program. The entire community was aware of the services and supported them. We mentioned that when a service station operator asked Mary Van Vactor, the PHN for the area, whether she had seen Joe Smith's wife, who was expecting a baby, Mary replied, "No." She then inquired where the Smiths resided. Soon she was on her way to visit the young woman on a small wheat ranch. When Mary arrived after a five-mile trip the woman greeted her with pleasure, happy to find that the two were acquainted through Mary's visits to the high school that Mrs. Smith had attended. They chatted. Mary asked how things were going on the ranch. Mrs. Smith seemed to be enthusiastic about her new life as a wheat rancher's wife. She volunteered the fact that she was looking forward to having a baby. Mary tactfully learned that the baby was due in about five months. She asked if Mrs. Smith had seen her doctor about her pregnancy. Mrs. Smith said that she had not, as they were very busy on the ranch, and that she felt fine. Mary explained the importance of prenatal care to preserve the health of both the mother and baby. Mrs Smith said that she would see Dr. Thompson soon. She did. Mary, knowing Dr. Thompson, called him and asked if he would like to have her visit Mrs. Smith occasionally. Dr. Thompson said that would be very helpful. Mary visited Mrs. Smith periodically during the next few months. She took her blood pressure, pulse, and weight, and discussed preparation for the delivery and for the new baby. In this instance, there were no complications. Mrs. Smith had a hospital delivery and after a week returned home. Mary again visited her, checked on the baby, and with Dr. Thompson's approval, arranged for the baby to be seen in the health department's well-baby clinic for physical check-up and immunizations. This was a real service for infants and pre-schoolers as the clinics were held in centers throughout the rural counties, quite distant from the Medical Centers.

In another instance, Mabel Spinning, a PHN, was helping in the STD clinic. The clerk came in and told her that a young teenager had asked to see her. Mabel greeted the young girl and ushered her into a small conference room. There the young girl burst into tears and sobbingly told Mabel that she and her boyfriend had been "sleeping together" and that she was afraid of getting pregnant. Mabel told the sixteen-year-old that the best way to avoid pregnancy was not to have intercourse. "But I love Tom," the girl replied. "Can't I take 'pills'?" Mabel arranged for the clinic doctor to see the girl. She had no evidence of STD but she obviously had been sexually active. Realizing that if the contraceptive "pills" were not provided the girl would undoubtedly become pregnant, the doctor prescribed the pills. Mabel explained how to take them and emphasized the importance of taking them regularly.*

I could relate many other activities such as arranging for and helping in the various health department clinics, giving immunizations, and making home visits to investigate possible communicable disease cases and contacts. The PHNs conferred with teachers on "teacher observation" for health problems of students. They made visits in the home to explain any abnormalities found in health screening exams of adults. They encouraged parents to have children examined by the families own physician. They helped make other arrangements as necessary. In addition, they made home visits on mental patients, prior to or after the patients had been seen in clinics or hospitals. They made many other types of home visits.

The major contribution of the PHN in providing preventive health services, as we have said, is made in the home. Mothers, particularly, and others have confidence in them. Often, as mentioned, valuable information is obtained in the home that otherwise would not be known. The PHNs are essential to the public health team. They have made major contributions to the preventive health services that we have reviewed.

This overall summary of health department services should serve as a means of evaluating those services, particularly as they might *relate to the demise of the plan for Local Health Units for the Nation. In making such an evaluation, we*

*In a similar instance, in another county, the parents learned that their daughter was taking contraceptive pills obtained from the Health Department. They arrived at the Department in an irate state threatening to sue. As Health Officer, I explained the situation and asked the parents how they would feel if their daughter became pregnant, after she had appealed to our department and been denied pills. They then calmed down. I discussed the matter with their family physician. He supported our action and conferred with the parents. We heard nothing further of the threatened lawsuit.

should be aware of the fact that the plan was never fully implemented. Had staffs been adequate and departments sufficiently financed, and were local health departments services extended nationwide, as envisioned, the record would have been even better. With this record of accomplishment, why have health departments not been better supported and expanded? Why has the emphasis changed from preventive coummunity health services to medical care and staff services been diverted from prevention to medical care?

Are there other possible reasons for the failure to support preventive health services of local health units as originally envisioned? If there are, what are they?

16. Failure of Leaders?

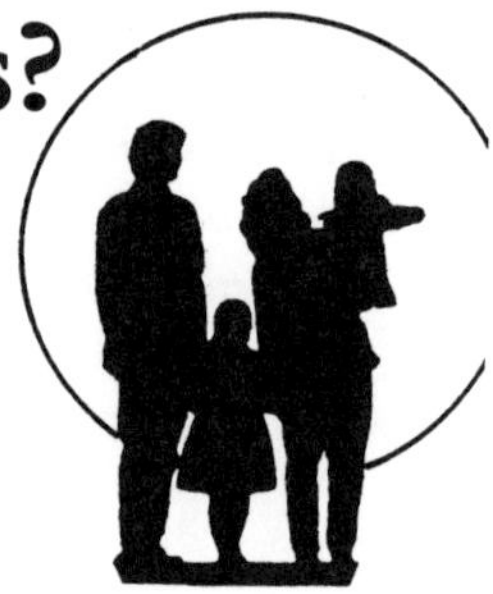

COULD THE FAILURE to implement the plan for "Local Health Units for the Nation" have been due to inadequacies in the leadership of health departments. Accomplishments under direction of able leaders have been reviewed.

In the late sixties and during the seventies, as many state boards of health were abolished, reorganization of public health services, with centralization of control of Health Departments in the offices of the President and Governors occurred. Qualifications of federal, state, and local Health Directors, frequently were changed to permit appointment of political supporters as directors, many of whom could not meet long established and proven standards. Losses of qualified leaders and deterioration of public health services began to occur. Health Department staffs were fragmented and many reduced. Some full-time Health Departments were abolished, and many were required to provide medical care at the expense of prevention. Leadership in many areas began to falter. In evaluating leaders, we need to ask several questions. Did these leaders recognize the public health needs of their communities? If they did recognize the needs, did they involve their staffs and their communities in evaluating problems and in planning to attack and solve them? Did they publicize problems and plans and obtain support of the medical profession, the media, and other influential groups and citizens? Did they acquaint governing and appropriating bodies with the problems and the value of Health Department services in better health and saving of lives, in addition to financial dividends which would result by investing in prevention? Did they communicate successfully with the Congress, with state, and with local governments on the problems, the plans, and on needs for financing? Obviously, some of the "leaders" left it to others to carry out these responsibilities!

Were some Health Officers content to mark time, to continue the same old programs without evaluating their results, or to get lost in the quagmire of medical care? Were they sufficiently interested in essential programs such as Mental Health and Environmental Health, or, were they satisfied in seeing essential elements separated from Departments? Did they motivate their staffs by involving them in planning and evaluation, keeping them informed on progress and successes, and crediting the staff for accomplishments? Did they bring the staff together as a team, or did they let the various units isolate themselves?

Were persons appointed to Director of Health positions who had little or no training in public health administration and who had little or no experience in public health? Were Health Officers appointed who were permitted to serve for insufficient periods of time to become acquainted with staff, public health problems and with programs under their jurisdiction?* Were terms of office too short to plan and evaluate progress and value of the programs? Did short terms preclude continuity of service? How frequently did political interferences and decisions negate sound professional judgements? Answers to these questions could determine how effective the leadership has been.

Is there a sufficient supply of qualified, Board certified, Public Health Physicians to assume leadership positions as Directors of State and Local Health Units?** Are salaries competitive? Have Public Health leadership positions been so politicized and leaders been so limited in promoting and developing public health services that such positions are no longer attractive? Do medical schools recognize the importance of public health and encourage students to enter the field. Are there a sufficient number of Health Departments qualified to offer good residency programs in Public Health? Whatever the reason, there is a critical shortage of well-qualified Public Health Physicians. Lack of these leaders is adversely affecting Public Health and the situation is worsening.

I would emphasize that there are many excellent Directors of Health Departments doing a creditable job. There are other capable Directors who cannot perform adequately because of limitations imposed by our revised political system and insufficient staff.

---

*Recent estimates are 2-2½ years average tenure for state Directors of Health.

**As stated earlier, in 1992 there were only 32 physicians in P.H. residency training in the entire United States!

Dr. Donald A. Henderson, Dean Emeritus, of the John Hopkins School of Health, on retiring as Dean, emphasized the "desperate need for leadership" in the public health profession. We can only conclude that inadequecies in leadership in some Departments in recent years have been a contributing factor in the breakdown of preventive public health services.

17. Excess Involvement in Medical Care?

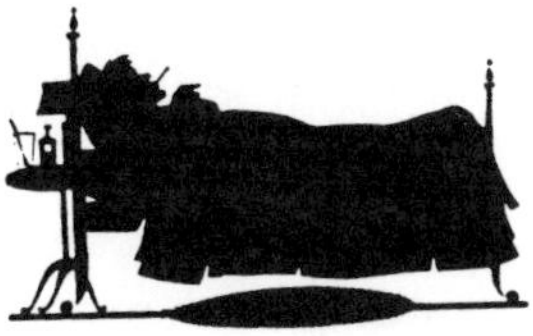

WHEN THE PLAN for Local Health Units for the Nation was first launched, the intent was primarily to control communicable and nutritional disease, to collect and analyze vital statistics, to improve maternal and child health, to improve maternal and child health, to improve sanitation and treat STDs to prevent spread. Primary prevention of disease and promotion of better health were the objectives. The medical profession, voluntary health organizations, and the general public were very supportive of these activities, and of the Health Departments.

Now the attention of government, many health agencies, the American Public Helath Association, Congressmen, Legislators, and others is focused on medical care over-shadowing prevention and community public health services.

Most everyone recognizes the need for a better system of medical care to assure good care for all. As some have said, we now have a non-system of medical care. Over 11% of our national income is spent for medical care. Unfortunately, financial support of preventive health services has declined significantly with less and less of our health dollar going for prevention (less than 3%).★ New programs, e.g. AIDS, Healthy Start, (for pre-school children), and Drug abuse control, and renewed efforts to control tuberculosis have been launched, but the infrastructure, the foundations for such services (Health Departments) have been neglected.

Many in public health and others, believe that Health Departments should be engaged in providing medical care, particularly for the homeless, and the many other poverty groups that make up the estimated twenty-five percent of the population that is not receiving medical care. Certainly there

★3% of a $540 billion health expenditure is spent on prevention.

is a need, but should Health Departments provide the care? Many Departments have been given the responsibility for such care, but there is question as to whether a Health Department can provide medical care and continue to do a good job in providing preventive health services.

In the 50's, Dr. John Kahl, then Health Officer of the State of Washington, firmly believed that his department could do a better job if it could provide both preventive service and medical care. He was convinced that they belonged together. He recommended to the Washington State Legislature that they transfer responsibility for welfare medical care from the Welfare Department to the Health Department. Dr. Kahl was recognized as an excellent administrator. He and his staff were enthusiastic about the change, thinking that this would be a real opportunity to provide a well-coordinated service.

Soon, Dr. Kahl found that he was having to sacrifice preventive health services in order to provide medical care. As medical care costs went up, he found that the Legislature would finance the medical care program but would not appropriate sufficient funds for the preventive health services. He was forced to divert staff from prevention to medical care. As he believed that prevention was equal in importance to medical care, and he knew that prevention had saved thousands of lives and millions of dollars in medical and hospital costs in Washington, after four years of frustration, and a heart attack, Dr. Kahl returned to the Legislature and asked that responsibility for medical care be given back to the Welfare Department. He did not want to see preventive health services sacrificed further.

During World War II, State Health Departments had a similar experience in the administration of the Emergency Maternity and Infant Care (EMIC) program. Assuring adequate obstetrical and infant care for families of servicemen was a huge undertaking which required expenditures far in excess of those previously made for community health services. Again, budgets for medical care were approved at the expense of preventive health services. This is typical of the syndrome of feeding the immediate need with no eyes for the future. Because the appropriations for medical care were insufficient to do an adequate job of administration, staff previously engaged in preventive services had to be diverted to help administer the care program. Health Departments did an excellent job in administering the Emergency Maternal and Infant Care program. The cost (about 10%) was low. There was no fraud, theft, or scandal connected with it. Many of us, however, welcomed the return to providing preventive health services.*

Individuals in Schools of Public Health, and many persons in official and non-official health agencies support more Health Department involvement in medical care. Unfortunately, as a result, preventive health services are often de-emphasized and neglected. Just as Fire Departments receive more recognition for putting out fires than for preventing them, so Health Departments are often given more credit and publicity for medical care and for controlling disease outbreaks than they do for prevention. A disease that does not occur seldom makes headlines! There is no question about the need for more and better medical care. The question is whether Health Departments should become involved in such care, at the expense of providing better preventive health services, or would the public be better served if they engaged in comprehensive, well-organized preventive services and left medical care to the private sector or other governmental agencies?

The trend to become more involved in medical care is another important factor in the demise of the plan for "Health Units for the Nation."

*Many illustrations of cost savings of preventive types of services can be given. The recent experience of the Sunbeam Corporation in reducing costs of obstetrical and infant care among their female employees is worth relating. Officials became concerned with the huge costs for such care (averaging $25,000 for each child born.) Many babies were being born prematurely requiring, in some cases, expenditures of $100,000 or more for care. Studies showed that many of these pregnant employees were not receiving adequate prenatal care. On instituting programs of health education, individual counseling, and prenatal care for all pregnant employees early in pregnancy, Sunbeam reduced the incidence of premature births dramatically and the average cost of obstetrical care of the mother and newborn infant from $25,000 to $4,000. The savings more than paid for the prenatal care programs.

This experience is only one of many that demonstrate what could be done if every pregnant woman was located and received adequate prenatal care. Again, demonstrations have shown the ability of adequately staffed Health Departments, cooperating with private physicians and hospitals, to assure such care on a cost-effective basis.

18. Inadequate Financing

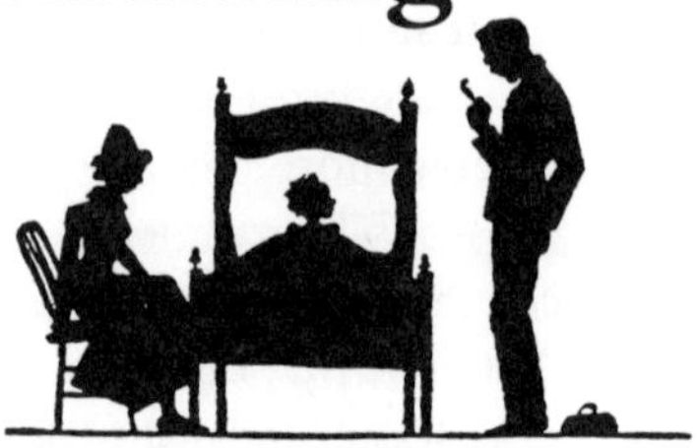

FINANCING IS ONE of the most important factors determining whether plans are implemented, or shelved. Too often good programs provided for in legislation are never or only partially implemented because of inadequate funding. This certainly has occurred in the case of Health Departments and programs. It has been interesting to me, and sometimes amazing, to see how very important decisions on appropriations for budget requests for programs vital to public health are made.

The procedures for obtaining funds have changed radically in the past fifty years. When I first had the responsibility for seeking appropriations, the manner was relatively simple. Our department prepared a budget outlining staff and salaries required, travel, supplies and other operating costs, and any requests for equipment. Without prior review by any intermediate body the budget request was submitted to a Board of County Commissioners similar to a Board of Supervisors. I made a personal presentation, answered pertinent questions and the Board usually approved the appropriation. The "carrot' of federal assistance made available through the State Health Department was very helpful. In Wasco County, the County Court (Commissioners) were reluctant to support much expansion in a new health department. In 1939, they were considering curtailment. Women's groups, particularly from rural areas of the County, appeared at the budget hearing and stated that they "received more service from the Health Department than from any other department of government" and that they wanted this service continued and strengthened. Their appearance was a spontaneous one and it was very effective. We had excellent data to present to the Commissioners showing that expenditures for Health Department services were an investment and resulted in savings to the County. Our budget was approved. That procedure was simple.

Believing that monies could be saved, many cities and counties employed administrative managers, officers, and budget analysts to assist them. Health Department personnel were required to be employed under a Merit System and a personnel classification and salary plan. Preliminary departmental budget requests were reviewed by a budget analyst, and presented to the County or City Administrative Officer for his or her recommendations. A total County budget proposal was then presented to the board.

The next step was for all Department Directors to explain briefly his or her department's budget to the Board and to answer questions regarding it. Support of advisory boards, conferences with individual supervisors in advance of the formal hearings, and appearances at the Board budget hearing were helpful in obtaining Board approval. Final action by the Board on the annual County budget was often deferred until the total estimated income and total budget could be reconciled. Sometimes the suspense was great. It also led to problems in trying to recruit staff and obtain supplies, space, and equipment for new programs. Dependence on state and federal funds as well as estimates on fees complicated the procedure.

In state government, the procedure for obtaining funds for health department programs became even more complex. In the twenties, thirties, and forties, the State Health Officer in most states, prepared a biennial budget request: presented it to a State Board of Health for review, and revision, or approval. In turn, this was presented to a State Budget Director, and to the legislature. As an example, in Oregon, as Health Officer, my staff and I prepared a tentative budget, taking into consideration public health problems, existing resources, needs for new staff, areas where problems had been solved and where cuts might be made. Program chiefs were given an opportunity to comment and help establish priorities. Occasionally a Governor, (Douglas Mckay was one who did), called state department heads together, briefly reviewed the financial status of the state with us and gave guidelines to use in preparation of a budget. Often this was not done by Governors. Governor McKay had been a very able businessman. He applied business administration policies to government. After review by the State Board of Health, the budget was presented to the State Budget Director. The first Director that I became acquainted with was George Aiken, in 1945. He was a "tight-fisted Scotsman." He reviewed our budget request in great detail, asked pertinent, incisive questions, and wanted full explanations and justifications for programs and particularly for new staff and equipment. He was reasonable in any deletions that he made and always explained the need for them. He had a staff of about ten persons to review all of the State Department budget requests.

The presentation of the budget to the legislature was the next step. The Oregon legislature had a Joint Ways and Means Committee made up of the Assembly Appropriations Committee and the Senate Finance Committee. To expedite its work, this Committee had a number of joint sub-committees, one designated as the Health and Welfare sub-committee. It had six to eight members. I was impressed with the interest that this sub-committee took in our budget. There was almost always full attendance and the hearing on our budget took many hours, usually requiring three or four sessions. Charts showing problems, programs, and progress were used effectively. After making our presentation, the sub-committee advised us of their action on each program, almost always approving as they had great confidence in the State Budget Director and the Governor. They knew that the budget was an "honest" one, that it had been carefully scrutinized and justified. Some program directors believed in presenting a padded budget with the expectation of reductions. With this strategy, I do not understand how a Director could sincerely or factually support it. To me, it would smack of Machiavellianism. In addition, legislators, and budget directors were astute in ferreting out padded items.

California had a different system. The Senate and the Assembly had separate finance committees, each with a sub-committee on health and related programs. Each sub-committee conducted its own review of the Health Department budget. (In California and in many other states, the budget was prepared and submitted by the Department of Health and was not reviewed by a Board.) Shorter presentations were made to the separate sub-committees, each allowed not over four or five hours. Presentations were duplicated. The Assembly sub-committee usually had for or five members in attendance. They primarily were interested in new programs, additional staff, and in major purchases of equipment. After each program, the Assembly sub-committee would act, generally approving the requested items. On the Senate side, however, it was quite different. Often only one senator, usually the chairman of the sub-committee, would be in attendance during the entire hearing!

After each new program had been explained, the Senator would say, "We will take that under advisement." I often wondered about a system which permitted one member to act for a committee, making decisions affecting the health of millions of people. We would learn later which items had been approved by the Senator. The two-committees then met in Conference. Generally the Senate version was adopted. Usually about half of our new requests were approved. The Senate Finance Committee and the Assembly Ways and Means Committee, the Legislature, and the Governor almost always accepted the Conference Committees recommendation. In California the Governor had the power to redline any item of which he disapproved.

Again, for reasons unknown to me, perhaps based on recommendations of the Council on State Government, the review system was modified. Oregon adopted the change two years after California. The State Budget Director's position was abolished and a Department of Finance was established. This Department with a Director, appointed by the Governor had a greatly increased staff. An analyst was assigned to work with one or more departments almost on a full-time basis. As at the county level, most of these analysts were very helpful becoming acquainted with public health problems, need for and use of staff, supplies, and equipment. Some, however, looked mostly at dollars and means of saving them, without enough consideration of the need for, and the benefits of a program.

I remember an analyst assigned to our department in Oregon. We invited him to sit in on three days of review of the budget by the State Board of Health. During the presentation, we explained the critical need for three child psychiatrists, a similar number of psychiatric social workers, and an additional clerk for our Child Guidance program. It was an excellent one. In the Mental Health section, we explained how a team of child psychiatrist, social worker, and clerk, traveled over the state conferring with teachers and parents and advising about children having psychological problems. The intent was to help the teachers handle most of the difficulties. Only the more complex problem children (and parents) were seen in the clinics and the teachers were often invited in to assure follow-up and to help them with similar cases. The need was great. Requests had been received from many communities that we had been unable to serve. Unfortunately, because of the inadequacy of salary and the necessity for considerable travel, one of the two budgeted psychiatrist positions was vacant. After the Board of Health review, I asked the analyst where he would reduce the budget request. He singled out mental health and said, "I would eliminate the request for all new staff in the Child Guidance program and

I would eliminate that vacant position of the child psychiatrist as it has been vacant for almost two years." Although the Board, composed chiefly of well-qualified professional people representing the public, had recognized the great need for, and had approved the request for additional staff, the analyst (only recently having graduated from college with a degree in business administration), overruled the Board. We did not lose the currently-budgeted positions, but we did not obtain approval for the new positions as the Department of Finance and the legislature accepted the advice of the analyst. I would have expected the analyst to ask why we had been unable to obtain the needed psychiatrist, and to offer his assistance in recruiting one. In his opinion, this would have cost more money and his objective was to save it. Mental health problems of children seemed to be secondary.

Lest I be mis-understood, I would emphasize that business managers and administrative assistants in state and local Health Departments are generally essential, and can be invaluable. Working as a team, such administrative staff insure that the dollars appropriated by the congress, the legislature, or a local Board, are effectively spent. Good business practices are vital in the successful operation of a department, I have been very fortunate in having some "top" administrative staff including fine secretaries. The State Board of Health could not have achieved the excellence of programs in Oregon without the dedicated services of Vernon Osborn, our business manager, Joseph Taylor, my administrative assistant, and many other devoted and able staff members.

To further consider the "changes" in budget reviews, many legislatures established "legislative analyst" positions with staff. These analysts acted as an arm of the Legislature and reviewed budgets as recommended by the Department of Finance and submitted by the Governor.

Apparently these reviews of budgets by Boards of Health, Departments of Finance, and a legislative analyst did not satisfy legislatures. Legislators, who formerly had had only secretaries to assist them, now employed additional staff, and most of the committees of the legislature employed staff to make further reviews of the budgets. These multiple reviews require considerable time of department's personnel as well as that of the reviewers. They really cost money! Considering this cost there is the real question of "savings" resulting from the multiple reviews. Trust in capable administrators seems to have been lost.

Inadvertently, special interest groups have competed with each other, and with general public health services, to obtain limited funds for public health. Congress frequently has responded by appropriating categorical, special, ear-marked funds to new agencies. The practice became so common that some labelled it as the "Disease of the Month Syndrome."

These funds have proliferated in number and have increased in size. In addition to funds for hospital construction, heart disease, mental health, and cancer control, Congress has supported categorical programs to combat many other diseases. There now are thirteen Research Institutes of Health, each established to control a specific disease, condition, or group of diseases or conditions, James B. Wyngaarden, M.D., who retired as Director of the National Institutes of Health in 1989, stated that one of his major problems had been in combatting special groups and congressmen who wanted to establish new Institutes. Such fragmentation increases costs and reduces effectiveness.

The Congress, state, and local appropriating bodies often fail to recognize that the potential for success of categorical programs cannot be achieved unless a basic service, the infrastructure, (Health Department service), is there to support it. One might compare the situation with a medical care system composed only of specialists. Without the services of a primary physician —a family physician or internist— to consider all of the needs of the patient, and, if needed, to refer the patient to specialists, good care cannot be assured. The primary physician provides the essential co-ordination of specialists care.

Categorical programs such as the ones to control the spread of the HIV and to prevent AIDS, to control tuberculosis and other communicable diseases, to provide pre-natal care, to assure good health care for all pre-school children, to maintain mental health and environmental health services, often are not co-ordinated, are duplicative, inefficient, wasteful, and are only partially effective. The major reason for this is because an adequately staffed Health Department has not been utilized to provide and co-ordinate the categorical services.

The diversion of funds from Health Departments to support separate "categorical agencies", is one of the reasons for failure to provide Local Health Units for the Nation.

19. Political Influence

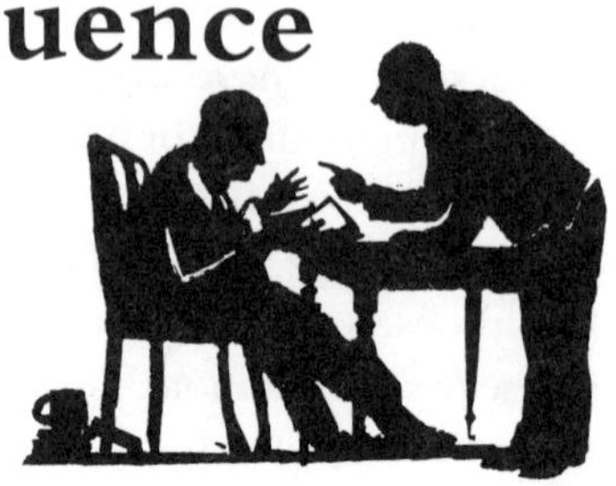

ANOTHER IMPORTANT INFLUENCE is that of Politics! How much influence has politics had on Public Health and Health Departments? Fifty years ago, most people would have replied "Of course politicians would not interfere with or over-rule professional judgements involving the public's health!" As community services developed, as special interests became more powerful, as the desire to control expenditures of large sums of money, and as varying opinions arose on how public health services should be administered and provided, politics became a major factor in the public health arena.

In analyzing this development, I will outline some of my observations and impressions on the increasing role of politics in determining the coursxe of public health services. I use the word "politics", not in the narrow sense of partisan politics and the influence of "Political Action Committees" (PACS). but in the broader sense, including the influence of leaders inside and outside of government. MY comments are based on observations made while intimately involved in public health administration during a great part of this century. I have seen the results of influences on public health by various political forces.

Public concern and efforts to influence congress and state governments began with private physicians who recognized the need for community action to control communicable disease. They realized that without an authority in government to enforce control, their efforts to prevent spread of communicable disease were rather fruitless. They organized, forming many state and local medical societties. (The American Medical Association was founded in 1847). Now, private physicans had a persuasive voice. One of their first major activities was to petition and request, by resolutions and by personal contacts and presentations, the Congress and state legislatures to establish State Boards of Health and Health Departments. Results did not come immediately, but with persistence, in many instances requiring several years of effort, many Boards of Health were established. It is noteworthy that in establishing these Boards, provisions were made in the law to minimize political patronage. Most of the Boards were composed of physicians, dentists, and pharmacists appointed by the Governors. Usually the members were appointed for four-year terms, on a rotating basis to assure continuity, and to discourage partisan changes by Governors. The Board, or in some instances, the Governor, appointed a Secretary of the Board to serve as State Health Officer. Further, the laws most commonly provided that the Health Officer be a qualified licensed physician specializing in public health and that his term of appointment continue two years after the beginning of a succeeding Governor's term of office. These provisions minimized political interference.

With major support from the medical societies, many local health officers were appointed as provided for in state law. As generally required in these laws, licensed physicians, qualified in public health, were employed.

These early Health Officers and Boards of Health explored problems of communicable disease and sanitation and applied control measures and measures for improving sanitation. After establishing procedures for reporting births and deaths, and the major communicable diseases, they implemented and maintained them.

The Boards were generally responsible for adopting regulations to clarify and detail provisions of state law. These regulations were adopted only after the public and concerned parties had been given an opportunity to be heard. It is significant that these Boards and Health Officers were given great authority to control communicable disease. They had authority to stop trains, to close harbors, and to quarantine ships. Many had police-type badges and some carried revolvers.

Full-time Health Officers were commonly dedicated, well-qualified physicians, selected because of thieř ability and interest in improving public health. They supplemented their medical knowledge and experience with experience in administering community health services. As public health schools were established and as physicians received graduate training in public health, including special courses in public health administration, many states amended their laws to provide that the State Health Officer, in addition to being a licensed physician and surgeon, must hav an advanced degree in public health. A further assurance of high standards for public health physicians was the establishment in 1949 of an American Board of Preventive Medicine and Public Health. This Board certified public health physicians who had received prescribed training in and who had qualified by examination. With a career ladder in the USPHS, superior qualifications of the Surgeon General of that service, and the high professional standards for State and full-time local health officers and health department staffs, very little partisan political interference in appointment of health personnel was possible. Merit System and Civil Service requirements in the expenditure of federal funds, administered by the Children's Bureau and by the USPHS for state programs, further minimized political patronage in Health Departments.

Using Oregon as an illustration, my predecessor as State Health Officer, Frederick D. Stricker, M'D., served for twenty-four years. He knew the state well and became very familiar with its health problems. Needed public health services were planned for with interested persons and organizations, and then implemented. Because of assured tenure, based on ability and performance, rather than on party affiliation or activity, he was able to develop and maintain continuity of programs. As a result, real progress in improving health was achieved.

At that time, continuity of service was assured in most all of the states. If a Governor was dissatisfied with the service of a Health Officer, he could, for just cause, have him removed by the Board. He could ask for the Health OFficer's resignation, or withhold salary increases from the budget, but he could not remove a Health Officer stricly on the basis of partisan politics and patronage, or make him a political scapegoat. Men like Dr. Chesley of Minnesota, Dr. Robert H. Hutchenson of Tennessee, Dr. Wilton Halverson and Dr. Malcolm Merrill of California, and Dr. Wilson Sowder of Florida, served under successive Governors for many years. They were "Career Health Officers", doctors thinking of the entire community as their "patient". Their records of accomplishment bear out the value of continuity of service of capable, experienced, well-qualified leaders. There were many others.

Authority to appoint and retain quality staff, based on training and experience, without political interference, was also important to the morale of staff and to the success of programs. Again, using Oregon as an illustration, during the perios 1945 to 1960, I served under seven Governors. Only once was I approached by a Governor or a member of his staff to appoint one of his political supporters. When the Governor called and asked that I appoint a particular individual to a vacant position, I told him that I appreciated his call and recommendation. I assured him that I could not think of a better reference for an applicant than the Govenor and that if the man qualified for the position in a competitive examination I certainly would be pleased to appoint him. Apparently this discouraged the Governor's friend as he did not apply for the job.

It seems that this provision for stability and high professional standards for key personnel was not acceptable to many Governors and political organizations. As we will discuss later, laws were changed governing the organization of Health Departments and the qualifications and methods of appointing State Health DIrectors and other staff.

A major influence on the scope and character of public health services was that of groups interested in specific dieseases. Illustrations of this type of influence are the actions of the national and state Tuberculosis Associations (Now Lung Associations) in promoting programs in Health Departments, and President John F. Kennedy's interest in mental retardation. Tuberculosis Associations realized that effective tuberculosis programs, except in rare instances, could not be effective without the services of a full-time Health Department.

Another area of citizen influence was in the field of sexually transmitted disease, (STD). In 1914, shortly after the establishment of the Children's Bureau, a group of leading citizens concerned with the serious illnesses and deaths resulting from syphilis, formed the American Social Hygiene Association, (ASHA). Charles W. Eliot, President of Harvard University, was elected to serve as its first president. This organization had considerable influence on the public, and later on the Congress. The American Social Hygiene Association carried on a widespread educational program on the incidence and hazards of venereal disease with particular emphasis on syphilis. It made studies of the incidence of prostitution and publicized the failures of cities to enforce laws prohibiting this practice. The APHA, the Association of State and Territorial Health Officers (ASTHO), and the AMA joined in petitioning Congress to establish a Venereal Disease Program in the USPHS. Congress did appropriate funds to establish national, state, and local programs to combat STD diseases.

Without the perseverance of its leadership and the continuing activities of the ASHA in encouraging national, state, and local governments to combat venereal disease, progress would have been delayed for many years.

The APHA was a unique organization. It was composed, initially, of national, state, and local public health professionals, health officers, sanitary engineers, public health nurses, sanitarians, vital statisticians, health educators, and other persons with a keen interest in public health. It established standards, carried on informal professional education, and served as a forum for discussion of community health problems and programs, and adopted policies and goals which it would support. During the early years of the Association, health officers played a dominant role. The Association concerned itself largely with control of communicable disease, improvements of vital statistics and laboratory services, development of local health departments, improving health services for mothers and children, and improving hospital facilities and other health services. It promoted the establishment of Schools of Public Health, and actually served as the official accrediting agency for these schools. It established standards for training, and qualifications of public health personnel. The major emphasis of this organization up until the early sixties, was on preventive health services. It promoted formation of local health departments. Through survey and development of plans such as Dr. Haven Emerson's "Local Health Units For The Nation", consultation to state and local governments by field staff represented by Dr. Carl Buck and other public health physicians, and supporting, national, state, and local public health legislation and appropriations, it had a great impact on the development and quality of state and local health programs.

On request, a state could obtain the services of the APHA to make an impartial survey of the state's health services and programs, to evaluate them, and to make recommendation for improvements. When I served as State Health Officer of Oregon, the State Board of Health requested such a survey. This was made in 1945 and the recommendations, which Dr, Buck suggested after several weeks of study, served as goals of the Board and were implemented during the next several years. Similar surveys were made in many states with similar results.

For years, the Association depended on Resolutions submitted to Congress, governmental agencies, or other policy making groups, to influence these bodies. Committee Chairmen, the Executive Director, or other key members of the Association occasionally presented Resolutions to committees of Congress and to other appropriate bodies. Such resolutions were of limited value, because the APHA had no representative in Washington, D.C. to present and follow up resolutions with members of Congress.

In 1954, I served as President of the Association of State and Territorial

Health Officers. Dr. Frank Yoder, State Health Officer of Wyoming, served as Secretary. We were responsible to the members of the Association to keep them informed on actions of the Congress on matters related to public health and to present the Congress policy recommendations as adopted by the Association. Dr. Yoder and I soon found that it was impossible for us to be adequately informed and to make timely presentations to Congress, not only because of the distance from Washington, D.C., but also because of our responsibility as Health Officers. We did not have the time to "bird dog" developments. We recognized that a representative of the Association was needed in Washington, D.C., one who could become acquainted with members of Congress and their staffs, who could present data and answer questions on public health when requested, learn of planned hearings on pertinent health matters, arrange for presentations at these hearings, and who could keep us informed. To finance such a representative would be expensive, but we agreed to explore ways of doing it.

I discussed the possibility of a representative for both ASTHO and APHA with Reginald Atwater, M.D., who was then Executive Director of the APHA. Dr. Atwater concurred in the idea and obtained the approval of the Executive Board of the APHA to explore proposals. Agreement was soon reached for the American Public Health Association, the National Tuberculosis Association and the State and Territorial Health Officers Association to employ jointly, Noble Swearingen as their full-time representative in Washington, D.C.. He served in this capacity for many years and was very effective. Actually, the State and Territorial health Officers Association had very limited funding but was able to participate in employing Noble Swearingen, through the assistance of a grant from another voluntary health agency.

For many years, the APHA was accepted as the major organization dedicated to improve preventive health services. In the early forties, this image began to change. The organizations began to take positions on social issues as well as on medical care.

Medical care did not become a major issue in the APHA until the early sixties. The physicians involved in public medical care programs and some staff members of Schools of Public Health, became increasingly concerned with inadequacies of medical care for segments of the population, particularly in the southern states. A medical Care Section was established in the APHA. Its membership soon surpassed that of the Health officers section, and began to dominate the organization. Although the Association continued its interest in promoting preventive health measures, its efforts in this area were diluted.

The ASTHO was influential because it represented the states and local communities in a partnership with the federal government to provide better health services for the nation. The relationship was a model for communication.

It is interesting to see how this functioned. Conferences with the Surgeon General of the USPHS and Chief of the Children's Bureau were held annually. The meetings lasted a full week. The Surgeon General and the Chief of the Children's Bureau (CB) addressed the Association, outlined problems and proposed solutions, discussed the status of public health legislation and appropriations, and presented questions on policy on which the Service wanted the advice of the Association. The USPHS and the CB recognized the wealth of experience of the State Health Officers and their knowledge of local needs and circumstances.

The Association had a number of committees including one on Federal Relations, and others on various public health program areas. These committees thoroughly considered the problems, and made recommendations which were then presented to the Association as a whole. All recommendations of the committees were carefully reviewed and discussed. Most were adopted. It was far from a rubber stamping process! The Health Officers were vitally interested in how changes in federal public health policy would affect their states. They were not hesitant in presenting their views! As Chairman of the Federal Relations Committee for many years, I have conducted meetings of the Committee which lasted into the small hours of the morning, with vigorous discussion. The recommendations, as finally adopted by the Association, were then presented to the Surgeon General and the Children's Bureau Chief, who did their best to implement the recommendations.

Health Officers not only noted the results of their recommendations through subsequent developments, but also through follow-up reports by the Surgeon General and by the Chief of the CB on each recommendation. These Conferences were very significant, often resulting in major changes in public health policy and services. A good illustration is the change in responsibility for the health services for Indians. This had been a responsibility of the Bureau of Indian Affairs. The Bureau had difficulty in recruiting physicians and was able to provide very limited health services for the Indians. State and Territorial Health Officers became concerned with the inadequacies and concluded that the USPHS could do a better job, particularly as it had a pool of career physicians that could be used to plan and to provide health services for Indians. It also had a good working relationship with state and local health departments. Dr. Albert Chesley, State Health Officer of Minnesota, led the "battle", and it was a battle! The law designating the Bureau of Indian Affairs as the responsible agency had to be changed. Year after year, resolutions were adopted and recommendations were made to Congress for the change. Personal conferences were held to enlist the aid of various Congressmen. Neither approach was successful. Dr. Chesley, with his well-worn and overflowing briefcase would not give up. The assistance of the APHA, prominent Indian leaders, and members of Congress was invaluable in bringing about this important change. Legislation was enacted in the mid-fifties transferring the responsibility for Indian Health from the Bureau of Indian Affairs to the USPHS. With its professional knowledge and other resources, with increased appropriations for Indian Health by the Congress, and with the cooperation of state and local health departments, health services for the Indians was markedly improved. The ASTHO took many other significant actions that resulted in great improvements in public health.

We have considered generally, how State Boards of Health were established and how some of the major health organizations that have had a major impact on the development of public health services have functioned. We have also referred to some of the voluntary health organizations that have had great influence on formation of Health Departments. To understand better how they influenced appropriations and legislation, let us consider some of the ways in which enactment of laws are initiated, and how legislative bodies are "lobbied."

In Congress, and in the states, bills must be introduced by Congressmen or by a Senator. Groups with special interests frequently persuade one or more of the members to sponsor a bill. The President or Governor may request one or more friendly lawmakers to introduce a bill or bills in which he or she had an interest. In many instances, departments of government recognize a need for legislation and initiate action to obtain it.

During the process of consideration, departments and representatives of the general public have an opportunity to present their views, either in committee hearings or to individual legislators. Private conferences with legislators or Congressmen can be considered lobbying. Those who do this are required to register as lobbyists, stating who they represent.

Legislators do need data and explanations and usually welcome them. To promote good relationships with Congressmen and legislators it is common practice to contribute to their election campaigns. Organizations that would lose their tax exemption status by engaging in politics often establish Political Action Committees (PACs), to which members of an organization contribute. Unions, Medical and Hospital Associations and other health organizations such as the AMA, sponsor PACs. Many organizations maintain headquarters in Washington, D.C., and employ lobbyists who reside there. The APHA, which for years had been headquartered in New York City, moved its entire staff to Washington, D.C., primarily to keep better informed on the activities of Congress, to get better acquainted with Congressmen, and to be readily available for Congressional hearings on health matters. Getting acquainted and working with staffs of committees of Congress often was found to be as important as working with Congressmen themselves!

Individual letters, cards, telegrams, petitions, calls, and other presentations to Congressmen, state legislators, and local legislative bodies also influence them and are frequently employed to support, or oppose, bills or measures that are being considered. Testimony before committees considering bills is important.

Two of the most effective presentations that I have witnessed in influencing legislation occurred in Oregon. A group of chiropractors, chiefly graduates of the Palmer School in Iowa, believed that chiropractic should be defined in law and that the practice should be limited to manipulation of the spine and joints. They were called the "straight" group. Two other groups of chiropractors, the "mixed advertisers", and the "mixed non-advertisers", were graduates of other chiropractic schools, one of the larger ones being located in Portland, Oregon. The "mixed groups" had sponsored legislation to require applicants for license as a chiropractor in Oregon to have taken courses in obstetrics, surgery, and on the actions of drugs. The basis was to "raise standards". Shortly after the legislature had passed the bill, the Governor had signed it into law, and the legislature had adjourned, the Attorney General ruled that because courses of study of obstetrics, surgery and drugs were required that chiropractors could now practice obstetrics and do minor surgery!

The "straight" group was alarmed. Although small in number, they raised funds for a "War Chest" to finance an attempt to amend again the Chiropractic Act, this time to limit the practice to manipulation of the spine and joints. Legislation was introduced and hearings were scheduled. On the day of the first hearing, bus loads of students from the Chiropractic School representing the "Mixed group", and others, packed the hearing room in the State Capitol in Salem. Most of these students were veterans of World War II. Their pleas to the legislative committee was that as they had fought for our country, and were enrolled in a chiropractic school, the scope of chiropractic should not be limited. Such limitations could jeopardize their future livelihood. The committee "killed" the bill.

A few years later, the "straight" group tried again. A bill once more was introduced in the legislature to limit the practice of chiropractic. The "mixed group" again responded by packing the hearing room. This time the chief and most effective witness was the young wife of a missionary. She obviously was in the last months of pregnancy. She testified that her two-year-old child had become ill while she and her husband were on a mission in the Far East. She stated that neither Japanese doctors nor an American Army pediatrician has been able to diagnose or treat the child successfully. She and the child had returned to Oregon. She said that she had taken the child to the chiropractic school in Portland for treatment. She testified, "they cured my child and are now taking care of me. One of their doctors will deliver my baby. Please do not deprive me of this wonderful service."

Although legislation was enacted which limited the practice of chiropractic in Oregon, defined minor surgery, and which prohibited chiropractors from prescribing drugs, it still permitted them to practice obstetrics! The packing of a hearing, and the emotional testimony of a few, can certainly influence legislation. Similar techniques are used effectively by many special interest groups.

Of even greater importance in influencing members of Congress and legislators are the activities of lobbyists. These individuals often represent special interests in influencing legislative bodies. These interests may or may not be in the best interest of the general public! Often the most effective lobbying is with legislative staff, and in contributing financially to election campaigns.

Enough on techniques. On with relating how politics has impacted public health.

A prime example of Congressional action resulting in break-up of Health Departments at the national level, and in many state and some local Health Departments, was the removal of responsibility for Environmental Health programs from the USPHS through creation of the Environmental Protection Agency (EPA).

Justifiably or not, Health Departments were criticized for failure to make progress rapidly enough. The critics failed to recognize the limitations imposed by appropriating bodies and courts.

Removal of responsibility for environmental health from Health Departments began with dissatisfaction and criticism of the the program, both from within and outside the USPHS. I served on President Eisenhower's Water Pollution Control Advisory Board and had an opportunity to observe and review the program being conducted by the USPHS, in cooperation with the states. It was excellent, considering the limited funds being made available by the Congress. (Just compare them with today's expenditures!) Cities were being cited for failure to treat sewage. Federal aid was being given to help build sewage treatment plants. Flagrant pollution of streams by industry, for example, the salt brine from oil industry operations was halted. Excellent research on environmental pollution control was being carried on. In retrospect, the failure to publicize adequately these successes probably was a mistake. The USPHS staff, largely made up of sanitary engineers, was doing a fine job,. There was an organizational problem. The engineers in the USPHS believed that their status in the Service should be elevated. This seemed reasonable. Water pollution control was an important function. It seemed to many that the water pollution control program should be one of the top level units in the Public Health Service. Requests fro reclassification of positions, and change in organization to accomplish this were made by staff. The requests were denied. Resolutions were then adopted by the ASTHO and the APHA to support the requests. Such appeals, made annually for several years were unsuccessful. Whether the Secretary of the HEW, the Budget Office, the Federal Civil Service, or the President and his staff were opposed, is not known but the sanitary engineers were finally convinced that up-grading in the USPHS would not occur. Not long afterwards, the Congress established the Environmental Protection Agency, removing the Water Pollution Control Program from the Public Health Service and combining it with similar activities previously carried out by the Department of Commerce, and other federal agencies. This gave much greater visibility to the program. Lawyers, in most instances, replaced sanitary engineers or physicians, as Directors of the new agency and its regional offices.

Many regional conferences on pollution and plans for control were held.

Appropriations for these programs were increased enormously by Congress. Whether the improvements in Environmental Health were proportionate with expenditures needs to be evaluated. Although some EPA officials have been accused of fraudulent practices, there is no question but what the environment has been given much more public attention since the EPA took over.

Again, the pattern established by the federal government was soon followed by many of the States. Several of them established State Environmental Health Agencies. Environmental health programs were often removed from State Health Departments and responsibilities for water supples, air pollution, and radiation control, occupational health services, restaurant, hotel, and other sanitarian activities were assigned to these new agencies.

Soon, counties in many states were making similar changes. Divisions or Bureaus of Sanitation were being removed from local Health Departments and the responsibility given to a new department or to another county department. This was proposed in 1973 in Riverside County, California, where I was serving as Director of Health and Mental Health. I explained to the Board of Supervisors that I considered the staff of the sanitarians and sanitary engineer to be an essential part of the Health Department. Sanitation was one of the prime reasons for establishing health departments. The participation of sanitarians was vital to many communicable disease investigations and their control. Sanitarians has always been included in our epidemiology teams. In addition, I pointed out that under the California State Code, recognizing health implications, the County Health Officer was responsible for the enforcement of over fifty laws in the sanitation field. As Health Officer, I could not assume the responsibility for enforcing these laws without authority to direct measures to ensure compliance. I further explained that the medical health officer has an important contribution to make in evaluating toxic wastes, radiation hazards, other pollution hazards, and in determining hazards to public health of various environmental conditions. Although many counties did remove environmental health from the Health Department, to the credit of the Riverside County Board of Supervisors, they retained the public health team, intact. This actual dissection of the Health Departments, removing an essential arm of the Health Department staff, is viewed by many as being very serious.

Failing to appreciate the results, this proliferation of categorical funds and programs, and the provision in enabling legislation permitting new, or agencies other than Health Departments to administer them, undoubtedly has been responsible for the continuing fragmentation of public health services. Confusion, lack of coordination, gaps in service, and inefficient use of funds have frequently resulted. This fragmentation is reflected in the service. Consider the family having a number of health problems. It could be receiving visits from a public health nurse, or aide, a school nurse, a social worker, a nurse representing Crippled Children's services, a venereal disease investigator, an AIDS Commission representative, a rehabilitation counselor, a sanitarian, and perhaps others! Now it is proposed that Tuberculosis Control workers be employed for follow-up in cases of tuberculosis. Each of these individuals is well-intentioned and has a common objective of helping the family. Too often these workers have heavy case loads and are unable to spend much time, if any, to look at the family as a whole. In many instances they check on one condition in one member of the family. Often they are not aware of the service of other agencies, or of other health problems in the family (or individual). Frequently, because of heavy case loads, the services are superficial.

Studies have been made in Great Britain that proved that when responsibilities for health and other social services were assigned to the one worker best able to serve the family and who could work intensively, spending sufficient time to consult with and help all members of the family, the results were far superior to fragmented service. Other workers provided specialized consultation and "back-up" for the "primary" worker. Perhaps we could learn from Britain's experience! Such fragmented service began to concern the public and government. In 1960, in California, Governor Edmund G. Brown appointed a select committee, the Governor's Committee on Medical Aid and Health chaired by Dr. Roger Egberg, which made a comprehensive study of governmental health services in California. In its final report the Committee stated, "Those needing health care are confronted by an uncoordinated multiplicity of professions, service agencies, and institutions. Federal, state and local governments have developed a series of unrelated health services to meet the special problems or needs of a particular group. Government agencies offer a patchwork of overlapping and piecemeal programs." The Committee further stated: "Health services must keep pace with California's growing population. Health services must also meet new needs and overcome new problems. The next fifteen years can bring to the people of the state either superior medical care and improved health, or a crisis of unmet needs, lowered quality care, and inflated costs." (Unfortunately, we now have a crisis.)

Another study made later in California by Dr. Leslie Corsa and Dr. Bruce Jessup, pointed out that in California, fourteen separate kinds of health services were being provided to half a million children. They stated, "Medical care for California's children provided from tax funds today is a confusing, fragmented jumble involving many agencies. Nowhere is it comprehensive and rarely is there reasonable consistency or coordination among the fragmentation." Chaos resulting from fragmentation is not peculiar to California. It exists to a greater or lesser extent in all states.

In an effort to coordinate health services, many states and local governments established inter-departmental committees to help bring about more uniform policies and improve services. These were of some help but did not solve the basic problem. Other states approached the dilemma through citizen groups. In Kansas, a committee of citizens developed a plan for Comprehensive Mental Health Services. The Committee recognized that official health services in local communities and areas needed to be improved for the "total person." It further recommended that a plan be developed "for the integration on a permissive basis, of local health and mental health services in a total community health service under one administrative director." This was further evidence of the widespread concern over the results of fragmentation and recognition that one health department could best serve the community. Unfortunately, this concept has not been a popular one as many more separate mental health as well as separate environmental health agencies have been established in states and local communities.

In an effort to coordinate health services at the state level, many legislatures enacted laws combining state departments concerned with health and welfare services into one overall agency, a Health and Welfare, or Human Resources Agency, paralleling to some extent, the federal program. California did this in 1961 combining several major departments including health, mental hygiene, social welfare, vocational rehabilitation, and the Office of Atomic energy development and Radiation Protection. Not only did many states establish such agencies but larger counties in many areas took similar action. The laws creating new agencies usually did not prescribe professional qualifications for the directors. The Governor, or other appointing authority, was authorized to select any individual who then served at his or her pleasure. In many instances those who were appointed did a good job. In others, the appointees were not qualified as administrators.

In California, a physician, who had no training in public health administration, was appointed as Director of the Agency by the Governor. One of the first statements of the new Director, as reported in the press, was, "I am not an administrator, and have had no experience in administration. I will leave administration to others in the agency!" Similar types of appointments have been made in recent years. Partisan politics has become more evident. Is the policy of "To the victor belongs the spoils!" in the best interest of the public?

As mentioned earlier, I served under seven Governors in Oregon. In earlier years, I was not aware of politics in appointments. The Governor and legislature appointed the officials and committees based on the interest and qualifications of individuals. The earliest evidence that I became aware of involving partisan politics in Oregon, was when Governor Paul Patterson, a Republican, failed to support appointment of Senator Robert Holmes as Chairman of the Committee on Education of the legislature. Senator Holmes had held this position for many years, and was well-qualified for it. When the change was made, it was strictly on the basis of partisanship. Understandably, Senator Holmes was angered. He ran for Governor at the next election and was victorious. When he assumed office, he supported primarily Democrats as committee chairmen. It is very evident that this type of practice not only prevails and occurs frequently at federal, state, and local areas of government, but that the general public apparently expects and accepts political patronage. These practices certainly have had a great influence on public health as well as other activities of government.

Dedicated career professionals, qualified through years of training and experience as leaders, often have been replaced by individuals "Loyal to the party," or by ones more likely to carry out the President's or Governor's wishes, irrespective of their merit. Although there are many fine people appointed to and serving in top administrative positions, too often we have lost the quality of experienced leadership and continuity of good service existing prior to political dominance.

Other victims of the political axe were the State Boards of Health. These Boards, made up of outstanding citizens who volunteered their time, served states well. Many of these Boards had functioned very effectively for over a century. The members were professional people: doctors, dentists, nurses, engineers, and pharmacists. Some of the State Boards had businessmen and other community leaders as members. These Board members were appointed by the Governor, usually on a rotating basis and for a specific term, to minimize the influence of partisan politics and the patronage system. Often appointments, were made from lists of names submitted by professional societies. Experienced and very valuable members were appointed repeatedly by successive Governors. Again, using Oregon as an example: Dr. N.E. (Steve) Irvine, served the state as a Board of Health member for over thirty years! All but the State Health Officer, and the Executive Secretary of the Board, served without pay! These Boards were not "rubber stamps." They established policy, reviewed budgets for the Health Department, and adopted regulations. They truly represented the public.

Suddenly, without reason, other than to centralize more power in the Governor and Directors of new agencies, states throughout the country abolished these Boards. In what respects did these State Boards fail to protect the public health?

Florida is a good example of a state that abolished its State Board of Health and of the serious consequences.

Disregarding the advice of the Florida Medical Association, that all community health programs should be in one health agency, using county Health Departments as the local operating unit, the Florida legislature in 1965, transferred the Community Mental Health Program to a division of Mental Health. In 1969, they abolished the State Board of Health after transferring responsibility for Air and Water Pollution Control and Narcotics program to another agency. An Ocald Star Banner editorial captioned "Board of Health is Dead," questioned the action, "When the State Board of Health had been doing such a fine job for the people of Florida." Later, the the Jacksonville Times-Union in a feature article called attention to the Board's eight decades of "proud history."

These and other similar comments had little effect on the Florida legislature. The change had been made. Problems with the re-organization were soon evident and party politics appeared in the health structure. Dr. Wilson Sowder who had served as State Health Officer from 1945 to 1969, now served as Director of a new Division of Health in the Department of Health and Rehabilitation Services. He was responsible to the politically appointed Secretary of this new agency. Dr. Sowder relates some of his experiences in his book, Florida's Health Under Eleven Governors, The Ins and Outs of It. To further illustrate, the new kinds of influence being encountered by many public health physicians , I quote Dr. Sowder, "Once I was pressured, for example, to give a license to a pest control operator who had failed the legally prescribed test we had given him. The matter was quickly dropped when I asked to have the order in writing. The Governor on one occasion began to admonish me severely for not closing two camps for agricultural workers in Dade County. Their shortcomings had been highly publicized. He stopped abruptly when I informed him that we, at the Division of Health, upon the advice of the Dade County Health Officer, Dr. Milton Saslaw, were in the midst of doing just that when our plan was vetoed by the Secretary of the new Department of Health and Rehabilitation Services, with written approval of the Governor's own office. I handed him the evidence. Members of his staff who were present then speculated as to what local political figure might have asked then to take this action. None of them could remember who it was, but the climate of opinion seemed to be that the action now appeared to be in a different light and quite proper since it had been taken for political, rather than health reasons." Dr. Sowder further states, "Efficiency suffered considerably under the new Department for many reasons, but mainly because the Directors were not allowed to perform even those functions permitted them under the new law. One day the Director of the Division of Administrative Services was lamenting to me privately the problems of the new Department. I told him to cheer up, that our efficiency had not been reduced by more than 20% under the re-organization. He was shocked at my estimate since it meant a loss of about $100 million worth of work each year for the state."

Apparently, problems became so great that the Florida legislature re-organized the Department of Health and Rehabilitative Services in 1975. Dr. Sowder reports that the re-organized Department "has not produced an even reasonably satisfactory health program, or maintained what we had before. The papers have been full of it, not sporadically, but constantly for the past three years." He also says, "Since annual reports were promptly discontinued under the new Department, it is very difficult for anyone to measure, monitor, or evaluate its work systematically and precisely."

Problems of the kind which Dr. Sowder reported on in Florida are not peculiar to that state. I have heard similar reports from public health physicians in many other states. On a visit to Berkeley, California, office of the Division of Health and Welfare Agency (prior to re-establishing the State Department of Health), physicians told me that they were severely handicapped in fulfilling their responsibilities because they had to wait for "almost daily instructions from Sacramento." There was no real delegation of responsibility. Effective programs were precluded, as the result of poor administration.

The political nature of many of the appointive positions is illustrated by an experience that I had when I came to California as Chief Deputy Director of Health. Firm in my belief that public health should be above partisan politics, I was registered as an Independent. Governor Edmund G. Brown personally assured me that public health should be non-partisan. I served as his appointee for many years. On one occasion I was requested to submit an undated resignation. I refused, but submitted a dated resignation. This brought an explanation that the procedure was merely "routine", and that my resignation was not wanted!

One of the more recent examples of political manipulation of State Health Departments Directors occurred in Pennsylvania in 1979. Gordon K. Macleod, M.D., who had been Professor, HealthServices Administration, at the University of Pittsburgh, was urged by the Governor Richard Thornburgh to accept an appointment as Secretary of Health of Pennsylvania. The State Health Department was sorely in need of revitalization. Fragmentation of responsibility for health services had occurred. After accepting the appointment, Dr. Macleod found within a few days, that there was no program of radiation control in the Department. It was in a Department of Environmental Resources. Mental Health, likewise was not a part of the Health Department. The Health Department had been stripped of a medical library and did not have as much as one book on Radiation Medicine! The Three Mile Island Reactor incident occurred about that time. Pennsylvania was faced with a possible nuclear disaster. Obviously, there was a serious threat to health. The State Health Department was immediately called on for help. Unfortunately, due to the fragmentation of health responsibility that had occurred, the State Health Department did not have the personnel or resources necessary to assist. Dr. Macleod did not hesitate to point out that "That there was little or no health input whatever in the many decisions made before, during, and after Three Mile Island." He recommended measures to strengthen the Health Department capabilities and to improve public health services. He testified before the Presidential Commission investigating the accident, expressing concern at the many deficiencies, particularly in public health, including mental health, which he believed existed prior to and during the incident. Shortly thereafter, the Governor called Dr. Macleod and asked for his resignation due to his public statements. Eight months after his appointment, as the news media headlined it "Pennsylvania Health Secretary Became a Three Mile Island Accident Victim." Dr. Macleod was concerned with community health, not with playing politics. Such political activity is much more widespread and is occurring much more frequently than it did in the past.

These changes have not been conducive to good health services. In many states, key personnel resigned or retired early. Morale of staff members of Health Divisions often suffered and public health services declined. In California, services became so poor that newspapers recognized the problems and publicized them. As a result of the public outcry, legislation was enacted to re-establish the State Health Department. In doing so, however, a State Board of Health which had been so effective and which had minimized political control, was not re-established. Another major omission was lack of qualifications for the Director. Previously, as we explained earlier, these were outlined in the law and provided that the appointee be a well-qualified physician-surgeon with special training and experience in public health administration. As only career public health physicians had this type of qualifications, selection of necessity, would be based on professional and administrative ability rather than on political affiliation. Without such a provision, public health physicians often were not considered for appointment to these important positions of leadership in health.

A similar situation has developed in the Health and Human Resources Agency. During most of our century, the Surgeon General of the USPHS was appointed from the career corps of USPHS Officers. He was responsible to the Secretary of the HHR and had considerable authority and influence. For the past ten years or more, physicians from outside the corps have been appointed as Under Secretaries for the health area. These physicians generally have been well-qualified physicians but several have found that their views are not in accord with the Administration and that often they have very little influence on policy. Realizing this, many have resigned. Depending on the administration, the Surgeon General was given more or less authority and at times had little visibility.

Surgeon General Julius Richmond made the positions of Surgeon general of the USPHS more visible. He again emphasized the importance of preventive medicine. Surgeon General C. Everett Koop did not have experience in, the knowledge of, or a real appreciation of the value of local health departments. He was the first Surgeon General of the United States Public Health Service to be appointed from outside the Corps. Surgeon General Koop was not a "Yes Man." He took forthright positions considering what he believed was best for the public rather than adopting what the Administration or special interest groups were advocating. his statements on the hazards of tobacco smoking, similar to those originally made by Surgeon General Luther Terry, his support of "free choice," although he was basically opposed to abortion, his declarations on "AIDS," and on "Driving While Drunk," captured the attention of the press, television and the general public. On these issues he did win the unofficial title of "Spokesman for the Nation on Public Health Matters." If he had focused attention on the inadequacies of preventive community health services and the need for Public Health Services For All, he would have had far greater influence on improving the health of our nation.

What the future role of the USPHS will be remains a moot question. There are those who are advocating abolishing it and replacing corps personnel with civilians. The proposal represents another illustration of political, special interest group influences on public health.

Can a distinguished service that has proven its value for over a century with a record of achievements in promoting and protecting the public health be abolished because of the selfish goals of a special interest group? We would hope not, but outstanding State Boards of Health with similar records of excellence were abolished!

After Reviewing the many political actions and results of pressures from within and outside of government, we must conclude that politics has been a major factor in bringing about the current chaos and crisis in providing good preventive public health services through Health Departments. Likewise, it has been a major factor in the abandonment or shelving of the Plan for Local Health Units for the Nation.

In thinking of re-vitalizing the Plan, we should again consider whether we need Nation-wide Health Units. Can we afford them?

20. Cost Effectiveness of Health Department Prevention Services

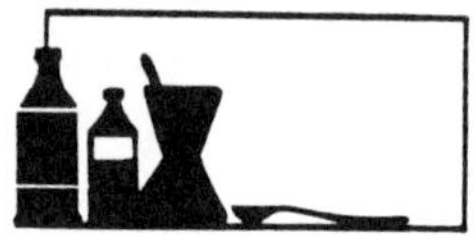

IS THE PLAN to provide Local Health Units for the Nation worth salvaging? Have the services provided in the past been cost effective?

A House Select Committee on Children, Youth, and Families reported that for every one dollar spent on immunizations, that ten dollars are saved in treatment costs. Another survey has shown that for every dollar spent by Medicaid on prenatal care, that over three dollars are saved in cost of care of prematures, infants with abnormalities, and mothers with complications at birth. The contribution of the Health Department in these cases is in finding the expectant mothers and in assuring that they are directed to good care. Physicians and clinics cannot provide essential care unless expectant mothers and others come for it! This help should not be limited to Medicaid recipients.

In discussing the communicable diseases in which Health Departments played a major role in control, the cost savings were tremendous. Think of the cost of care of paretics—those with syphilis of the brain—who occupied 10% of all State Mental Hospitals in the early forties. This was only a small part of the cost of care of all persons contracting syphilis. Health Departments were effective in tracing contacts, in finding new cases early, counselling them to limit spread of the disease, and in getting them under treatment, again with great savings.

Imagine the cost of hospitalization, when required, and medical treatment of patients with tuberculosis. When the disease was widespread, states and counties maintained large hospitals, sanitaria, and pavilions for patient care at huge expense. Health Departments played a major role in earlier control of this disease.

Similar statements could be made about polio, diphtheria, and other communicable disease.

The occasional outbreak of salmonella, staph food poisoning, botulism and waterborne disease emphasize the value of preventing them.

Screening programs to find children early with physical and developmental defects, to find children who have not had protective immunizations, and to assure that parents understand the need for care and arrange for corrections or treatment, do save and could save a great deal more if Health Departments were adequately staffed.

Voluntary health agencies, hospitals medical auxiliaries, and Health Departments often conduct screening programs for adults. The intent is to find individuals with cancer, heart disease, high blood pressure, diabetes, cataracts, glaucoma, hearing losses, arthritis, and similar conditions. These programs are valuable but too often the necessary follow-up to insure that the individual with a problem understands it and seeks more specific diagnosis and treatment is overlooked, is inadequate, or is not done. Health Departments, where organized and with adequate staffs, can provide this valuable follow-up service but often are not called on.

Adequate follow-up to assure that community facilities are available and that needed treatment is being received by patients discharged from State Mental Hospitals or who otherwise would be in Mental Hospitals has saved millions of dollars. More important is that it restored a quality to life for hundreds of thousands of people. Unfortunately, because these community services are either non existent or totally inadequate due to insufficient funding, too many individuals become a part of the homeless population or barely survive.

Programs such a methadone treatment for heroin addiction, alcoholic rehabilitation, and support programs for those addicted to cocaine and "crack", although far from being adequate, definitely have saved communities millions of dollars in decreased crime and government support. Regretfully, many of these savings are not obvious immediately. They are long-term and, therefor, are frequently over-looked.

To put a value on conditions that do not occur, on prevention, is difficult, but even a superficial evaluation supports the old proverb, "An ounce of prevention is worth a pound of cure!" This is applicable to communicable disease control or pre-natal care, protective immunizations for children, disaster preparedness, and other preventive health services in which Health Departments are involved.

Community preventive health services have proved to be cost-effective!

21. And What Of The Future for "Local Health Units for the Nation"

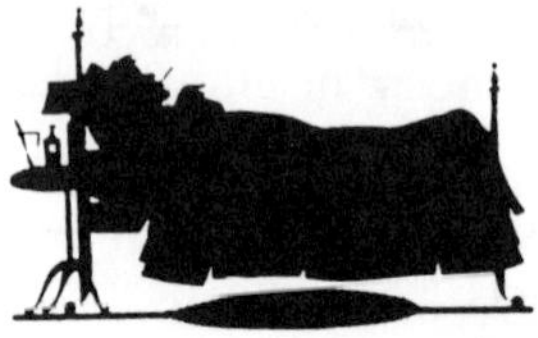

IS THE PLAN unrealistic? Are public health services now so fragmented that only a massive re-organization and consolidation could restore an effective program? An impartial evaluation would show that the Plan was sound. As we have seen, the departments that were established, although understaffed, made a major contribution to the public's health with preventive community health services. Why weren't they given greater support? We have reviewed a number of possible reasons. Was it one of them, or a combination?

We constantly hear that prevention is important, but we continue to expend more for medical care and proportionately far less for prevention. Community health services for prevention are essential to any health program intended to reduce illness, accidents, and unnecessary deaths.

At a recent Summit meeting on Education, the Governor of New Mexico in a closing session said, "Give us a healthy child and we will provide a good education for that child." We are giving a great deal of emphasis to the need for improving education, and rightfully so. The assurance of good health is equally important!

The deficiencies in public health programs and the chaos in providing community preventive health services is acknowledged and recognized widely. There have been a Summit meeting, major studies, conferences, and other meetings to consider the problems.

The Department of Health and Human Resources which called the Summit meeting, issued a report, "Healthy People 2,000—Year 2,000 Health Objectives for the Nation." The Institute of Medicine, after much study, issued a report, "Future of Public Health." The American Public Health Association Executive Board has proposed the "APHA Target for the 90's." The American Medical Association recently re-affirmed its support for "Local Health Units for the Nation." The communicable Disease Center has stated its goal to "Improve the Public Health System."

The targets, goals, and objectives for improving the public health are excellent but the most important question on how we reach them was either not considered or unanswered. The Institute of Medicine concluded that Public Health is a vital function that is in trouble, and urged readers to get involved in their communities. The American Medical Association's support of local Health Departments is the only specific suggestion that would help in reaching the stated, goals, targets, and objectives.

Realistically, if we are to ponder a plan to reach the goals, out lined, we must consider some vital questions:

1. Do we need a plan to organize and re-vitalize community preventive health services?

2. Do we need to co-ordinate existing services to eliminate duplication and gaps?

3. Do we need to designate one agency to have prime responsibility for implementing a plan for developing, maintaining, and coordinating a program?

4. Could the dollars now being spent, the many professional activities being carried on, and the un-coordinated efforts of multiple agencies to control single diseases, and to serve isolated segments of the population, be more effectively used if they were consolidated, organized, or coordinated to meet all of the public health needs of families and individuals?

4. What incentives might be offered to agencies to co-operate in making changes?

5. How could a revised programs be financed?

The need to develop a plan to resolve the present chaotic state of public health is of such importance that another Summit meeting should be arranged to make specific suggestions on how the goals and objectives of "Health People 2,000" and recommendations of the Institute of Medicine might be attained.* Representatives of organizations (governmental and non-

*Another conference entitled, "Healthy Children, Ready to Learn: The Critical Role of Parents," was held in February 1992. It was sponsored by the Office of the Surgeon General, Antonia C. Novella, M.D., M.P.H., other governmental agencies, and the National Governors' Association. The Conference recognized that children are the nation's single greatest investment in the future, and that their needs must be met.

The roles of health professionals and parents were emphasized. Ideals for health care of children and youth were outlined. These were excellent but again, realistic plans to achieve the goals, the "how", were not established.

governmental) participating in the 1st Summit meeting should be invited. It is essential that the White House and Congress, associations and agencies currently having a responsibility for public health services or a vital interest in them, be represented. These would include; the Association of State and Territorial Health Officers; Associations of City and County Health Officers; American Medical Association; national associations of dentists, public health nurses, Schools of Public Health, and Medical Schools; the American Public Health Association; the Academy of Preventive Medicine; the American Association of Public Health Physicians and the "Partnership for Prevention."

If participants in the "Second Summit" could agree on a realistic "plan" to take us out of the current morass and to establish a nationwide effective public health program, a major advance would have been made towards the established goals. With a commitment of each of these delegates to enlist the full support of the agency or organization which they represent, implementation of the "plan" could be achieved.

In developing this new "plan" we could benefit from previous experience by reviewing the development of and the early successes of local Health Departments. There was a Plan. Congress designated the U.S.P.H.S. and the Children's Bureau to implement it. Funds were allocated for use by the states in establishing new local Health Departments and strengthening existing ones. Funds were made available for training public health professionals, through grants to schools of Public Health. Students were offered stipends. Financing for Demonstration Projects was made available. Standards for P.H. personnel were established and merit systems were required to preclude employment of unqualified individuals. Although public health problems were similar in most areas, much flexibility was permitted to best attack them. The progress in implementing this "Plan" was impressive until World II disrupted it.

The initial "Summit" has resulted in some developments that have promise. "The Partnership for Prevention" was organized in the private sector to ensure emphasis on prevention in national health policy. The intent is to help implement the recommendations of "Health People, 2,000". This organization has broad membership including consumer groups business, industry, Universities, and professional and trade associations. The original Chairman, Honorable Richard Scheweiker is President of the American Council of Life Insurance. Honorary Co-chairmen is Mrs. Albert Lasker.

A Western Consortium for Public Health has been established. C.D.C.

selected this consortium for a co-operative program to develop and conduct a "Public Health Leadership Institute." This is a one year's scholars program for Senior State and local Health Officials from throughout the United States.

The Communicable Disease Center (C.D.C.) has stated a goal "to improve the public health system."

In developing a new plan. Health Departments with their earlier records of success, as we have reviewed them, would seem to be the agencies to be selected to be re-vitalized and to have a major role in a new coordinated prevention oriented community public health program. There are other alternatives. Health Sciences Universities with their medical, dental, nursing and other health personnel and students, have stature and favorable access to funds. Many could establish local centers (some have) and develop community public health services. Many now administer Crippled Children's services. Departments of Education have a major interest in the health of school children. They, too, have great financial support. Many have school nurses. Some employ school physicians. They have rapport with parents. They are not embroiled in medical care. Perhaps they could expand their health services with home visits, locating and assuring pregnant girls and women of good pre-natal and post-partum care. Immunization of infants and preschoolers could be provided. They could develop other needed P.H. services.

Schools of Public Health, like-wise have the expertise and if adequately financed, in some areas, might develop preventive public health services.

Another resource that has been suggested and might be explored is a non-governmental contractual agency. One of these or perhaps a combination of them are possibilities for providing the needed services.

Whatever the agency, essential elements in it should be a well-trained staff with the needed support services, good morale, an able well-qualified leader and director, freedom form political interference and good liaison with private physicians, dentists, other health professionals, and hospitals. The support of the community and good rapport with the families and individuals served is a basic necessity. A sound relationship with both government and volunteer agencies is like-wise very important.

In many areas of the country, local Health Departments have operated quite effectively for many years and have most of the requisites. We have previously discussed their activities and successes. Recently, most have been burdened with medical care and have inadequate staffs being particularly short of public health nurses and aides. As a result, they have not been able to render the kind of preventive health service they are capable of. It would seem that the best way to provide nation-wide preventive health services would be to build on existing Health Department infra-structures. These departments would need to be re-vitalized and adequately staffed. New Health Units would be required for those areas currently without the benefits of them.

We have some excellent models of good Health Departments that have been adequately staffed with proven results. These should be expanded and tried on a much wider basis. The best model of total health care that I am familiar with was the medical program conducted at an "atomic" city, Hanford, Washington. It was a part of the General electric Atomic Energy program. Dr. William J. Norwood was Medical Director. Dr. Ralph Sachs was Director of the Health Department.

The feature of the program that was unique was the outstanding coordination of preventive health activities with medical, surgical, obstetrical, and hospital services. Costly duplication of effort, of hospital and related facilities, x-ray and other laboratory services, and of health records was largely eliminated. The staffs shared adjacent office and clinic space. Public health nurses visited families in their homes. They did follow-up on patients referred by physicians.

Reports were given to the physician and joint records were maintained when indicated. The public health nurses did counselling, made contact investigations, screened for women who needed prenatal care and arranged for that care. The Health Department, the hospital, and the medical staff cooperated in screening for early health problems. Together they conducted pre-employement examinations and health education programs, did disaster preparedness planning, and implemented a complete health program. Referrals between , physicians and Health Department personnel were freely made. Conferences and notes on common records helped assure a high quality of service.

The industrial health program incorporated in the overall program resulted in one-half the absentee rate of comparable industries. The resulting savings were sufficient to pay for the entire industrial health program! Employees had been recruited from every state and from all walks of life. Many of them were handicapped.

A five-year study begun in 1944, showed that death rates in the "atomic city", when corrected for age differences, were one-half of those for the

United States as a whole. Morbidity rates likewise were considerably lower. Dr. Norwood reported on this program in the Journal of the AMA in the issue of January 2, 1954.*

Another program that could be used as a model was that of Wasco-Sherman Counties Health Department in Oregon, created when Health Departments were first being established. The Department was small, but so were the rural counties with a combined population of about 15,000 residing in an area of over 3,000 square miles. The staff was composed of a full-time physician, five public health nurses, a sanitarian and a clerk. Except for treatment of STD, the Department offered only preventive health services. It cooperated very closely with the local physicians, the two hospital staffs, and with the only voluntary health association, the Wasco County Health Association. The most valuable service of the Department was that given by the public health nurses (PHNS). They visited the homes considering the health status of all members of the family. Home visits included follow-up on health screening programs in the schools. They did the vision and hearing testing in the schools and health Department well-child clinics. Emergencies in the schools were handled on an "on-call" basis. The Department did quite thorough physical examinations on new students, entering school children, and on high school seniors. Patterning after the teacher screening program developed in Astoria, new York, they counselled with the teachers on "teacher observations" for health problems and arranged for school physical exams for those needing them. Referrals for care were made to the family physician or physician of choice, after conference with parents either in school or in the home. Those PHNs had a wide acquaintance with the school children, and with families. They actually learned of every expectant mother and infant in the two counties.

The Department conducted many clinics including well-baby, preschool, immunization, tuberculin testing, and STD clinics. The sanitarian did an excellent job checking on water supplies, dairies, restaurants, waste and sewage disposal, and in rodent and insect control. All Health Department services were available to any person in the Counties without charge. This was based on the premise that these tax-supported preventive community health services, like education, actually benefit everyone.

The results of the Health Department programs were dramatic. In three years, infant mortality rates had dropped by over sixty percent! Stillbirths

*A.M.A. Jan. 2, 1954: V 1543:44-49. Copyright 1954, American Medical Association.

fell by fifty percent. The reduction in reported cases of tuberculosis, typhoid fever, smallpox, syphilis, and other communicable diseases was striking. Although based on a small population, the declines were unquestionable. The value to infants and children in finding abnormalities and obtaining corrections or treatment was huge. Cleaning up public water supplies, dairies, and restaurants was invaluable.

Residents of the counties were thrilled when they heard Sam Hayes, broadcasting from San Francisco in April, 1940, say, "Hats off to Wasco County, Oregon, for their splendid Health Unit!" Wasco County has won first place in the Western Division (Comprising eleven states and including Los Angeles, California) of the 1939 U.S. Chamber of Commerce sponsored Rural Health Conservation Contest. The residents of the county, and particularly the physicians, deserved the credit for supporting and cooperating with the Health Department.

Another department that has an excellent program whose director has received national honors is the Palm Beach County Health Department in Florida. Dr. Clarence L. Brumback, Director for over thirty-five years, received the Sedgwick memorial Award of the APHA for his record of achievements, particularly in the fields of environmental control, maternal and child health, and immunizations. Many health officers have stated that this Florida County Health Department could well serve as a model for other departments.

A state program for support of county public health services worth emulating is that of California. It has done a better job of supporting local health departments financially and in providing basic preventive health services for more rural counties than most other states. The "contract counties" receive good quality basic health services on a partnership basis with the state. The county employs public health nurses, sanitarians and, in some areas, a health educator. These usually are recruited for the counties by the state. The state provides consultation and supervision by public health physicians, sanitary engineers, sanitarians, public health nurses, and health educators. The state also provides more populous counties with state funds to help maintain full-time Health Department service. This program has been very successful. although funds in recent years have not kept pace with the needs. Funding of medical care programs now has taken precedence over prevention, resulting in very inadequate funding of preventive public health services.

Undoubtedly, there are many more Health Departments that have provided outstanding services and that could be used as models. The key elements of success in these programs were; good leadership (in the programs cited, these were physicians trained and specializing in public health); having sufficient staff and facilities to provide the services; cooperation between the physicians and the Health Department; mutual trust; free exchange of information; and two-way referrals between them. Public understanding and support were essential.

What is the possibility of providing similar services nationwide? That would depend on a resurgence of interest in the Congress, in the states, and particularly with the public in having a nationwide community health service for prevention, and a comprehensive network of Health Units. The public would need to be made aware of the Plan for such service, the critical need for it, and of the fact that such a plan has never been implemented. The public should know of the shambles that community public health services are now in, of the inadequacies of our Health Departments and of the need for a protective public health net to help in the control of epidemics such as AIDS. It should know that public health services are almost non-existent in many areas or our nation and in most, they are so fragmented that effectiveness of service is almost impossible to evaluate.

How might renewed interest be aroused? Conferences, Commission Studies, annual sessions of national organizations and meetings to discuss the needs for better preventive health services are helpful. As mentioned earlier goals and targets have been established, but unfortunately, no plan has been developed to reach them. A sound plan for massive organization and action, with inspired and dedicated leadership to implement such a plan, is needed.

If the American Medical Association, that initially was so effective in promoting the establishment of Health Departments, if the American Public Health Association, The American Dental Association and member organizations of the Coalition that sponsored the 1990 Conference on "Prevention," joined in, informing their members of the need for assuring a nationwide, comprehensive, health service for prevention and lobbied for it; if leaders of Congress who have expressed concern about public health could be motivated to develop or support a plan like "Local health Units for the Nation" and who would mobilize congressional support for the plan and the funding of it; and if wide-spread public support was demonstrated by large numbers of letters, telegrams, calls, and conferences with Congressmen; then and only then could such a plan be implemented.

Special interest groups now promoting fragmented programs would need to recognize that without a firm foundation of basic health department service, specialized preventive health services cannot be effectively and economically provided. They would need to support the plan.

Support of the media would be essential in a campaign of this magnitude. Similar campaigns would have to be mounted in the states and in local communities. Such a program is not impossible, but, as has been said, it would require aroused public support and dedicated leadership to accomplish it.

This leadership must be found and supported in our highest levels of government, national, state, and local. Leaders, convinced of the need for preventive public health services for the nation, must arise in public health itself, to meet the challenge. Again we must heed the admonition of Dr. Donald A. Henderson, stated when he served as Dean of the John Hopkins University School of Hygiene and Public Health: "We must face the fact that the public health profession is more desperately in need of leadership than perhaps any other sector of society."

Although there are some excellent leaders, few, if any, are promoting a plan for "Local Health Units for the Nation." We are paying the price of ineffectiveness of many in leadership positions, and for the inadequate numbers of effective leaders, as discussed in the section on the crisis in Public Health. In the past, leaders have emerged to face such a crisis. They must do so again. The future of essential preventive public health service for all of our citizens is dependent on it.

References

The United States Public Health Service, 1798-1950, Ralph C. Williams, M.D.

Shadow on the Land, Surgeon General Thomas Parran, U.S.P.H.S.

Journals of the American Medical Association, as referenced 1905, 1906, Atomic City: W. Daggett Norwood, M.D.

A.M.A., Jan. 2, 1954: V 1543:44-49, Copyright 1954, American Medical Association.

Mortality and Morbidity Statistics 1940-1991, National Center for Health Statistics, Centers for Disease Control.

Center for Disease Control

Morbidity and Mortality Weekly Reports-Summary

National Center for Health Statistics and C.D.C.

About the Author

HAROLD M. ERICKSON, SR., M.D., M.P.H., graduated from the University of Oregon Medical School in 1933. He completed an internship and was the first resident in pediatric surgery at Doernbecher Memorial Hospital for Children in Portland, Oregon. Leaving private practice, Dr. Erickson accepted a position in The Dalles, Oregon as the first Director of Health of Wasco (and Sherman) counties. He developed a Health Department program that won a U.S. Chamber of Commerce Award in 1940 as the best on the Pacific coast.

Witnessing the dramatic results of preventive community health services in the control of Small Pox, Diphtheria, Tuberculosis, and Syphilis; other communicable diseases; in the marked reduction in maternal and infant deaths; improved child health; and in better sanitation, he elected to continue in public health. He obtained a Masters degree in Public Health at John's Hopkins University and returned to Oregon as Director of Maternal and Child Health. He was appointed Assistant, and in 1945, State Health Officer of Oregon. During his fifteen year tenure, Oregon established the first Air Pollution Control and Radiation Control programs in the United States. A Medical Examiner System replaced an Antequated Coroner System. Oregon achieved the lowest infant and maternal mortality rates in the United States for one year.

In 1960, Governor Pat Brown appointed the author as Chief Deputy Director of the California State Health Department. He resigned in 1966 to accept a position with the Ford Foundation as a Consultant on Family Planning to the Government of India—Punjab and Haryana States. In 1969, Dr. Erickson became Director of Health of Riverside County, California. He developed the County's first Community mental health program which became one of the fore-most in California.

Dr. Erickson has served as an Assistant Professor of Public Health at the University of Oregon Medical School and Loma Linda University School of Public Health. He has been a guest lecturer at the University of Minnesota and at the U.C.L.A. School of Public Health. The author has served on many national and state commissions, boards, and committees. He has published a number of articles on public health.

The author was appointed by President Eisenhower as one of three U.S. Delegates to the World Health Assembly in Geneva, Switzerland in 1954, and to the President's Water Pollution Control Advisory Board. He was President of the State and Territorial Health Officers Association and of the American Association of Public Health Physicians. He is Life Member of the A.P.H.A., member of the A.M.A. and affiliates, the College of Preventive Medicine, and the American Association of Public Health Physicians.